NUTRITION
FOR MARATHON
RUNNING

'An empty sack won't stand up'

Old African saying

NUTRITION FOR MARATHON RUNNING

JANE GRIFFIN

THE CROWOOD PRESS

First published in 2005 by
The Crowood Press Ltd
Ramsbury, Marlborough
Wiltshire SN8 2HR

www.crowood.com

British Library Cataloguing-in-Publication Data
A catalogue record for this book is available from the British Library.

ISBN 1 86126 590 5

Acknowledgements
To my husband Chris for his love as well as his patience and support
– again!
To my children Daniel and Jessica for their love, interest and
encouragement.
To my brother Robin for sound advice.
To the thousands of marathon runners I have met whose questions
about diet inspired me to write this book.

Typeset and designed by D & N Publishing
Hungerford, Berkshire.

Printed and bound in Great Britain by Biddles, Guildford.

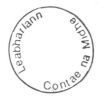

Contents

Introduction

You may have picked up this book because you are thinking about running a marathon, have already started training for your first marathon or have run one that went very wrong. Your motive for running 26.2 miles may be to lose weight, generally get fitter and healthier, or raise money for charity. Perhaps you were inspired watching Tracey Morris run and win her first marathon at the 2004 Flora London Marathon and then go on and finish twenty-ninth out of eighty-one starters in the Women's Marathon in the Athens Olympics. Whatever your reasons, I hope this book helps you to achieve your personal running goal.

Evidence continues to mount on the benefits of physical activity for the well-being of body and mind. The protective effects are as strong as not smoking and include reduced risk of heart disease, cancer, diabetes, osteoporosis and, of course, overweight and obesity. Regular running may help you cope better with the daily stresses of life and promote healthy sleep patterns. The running body is like a high-performance car. You would not use low-grade petrol and oil in such a car. You would not neglect to top up the battery or keep the tyres at the right pressure or the bodywork clean and sparkling. Similarly, the running body needs the right foods and fluids to provide energy and all the essential nutrients to keep the muscles and nerves functioning efficiently, the joints supple and flexible, and the body well-hydrated.

This book has a brief introduction to nutrition and then explains how the running body works. The next two chapters give practical advice about what, when and how much to eat and drink to maximize performance. Chapter 4 helps you to prepare for the marathon itself, including giving the low-down on carbohydrate loading, how to manage water stations efficiently, and what to do in the days after the marathon. After a short chapter on ergogenic supplements (things that may or may not help you to perform better), the next chapter covers specific issues you need to consider if you are a vegetarian, female, veteran, diabetic or a wheelchair marathoner, or if you are planning to run a marathon in a cold or hot climate. Finally, 'Running into problems' gives advice on dealing with certain difficulties that you hope will not happen.

When I ran the London Marathon, in 1986, at about 20 miles I encountered one of these difficulties. A huge amount of my training had been done in the evening and none before midday. My body was stunned by the early start and, although my legs knew what to do, my gastrointestinal system was totally confused. Accessible loos were few and far between. On a positive note, I have the marathon to thank for my husband's interest in cooking. As my Sunday training runs got longer and longer, my children were in pyjamas before Sunday 'lunch' was ready. So Chris took over and to this day still cooks our Sunday lunch. Happy running and happy eating.

Jane Griffin, Sports Dietitian and Nutrition Consultant

CHAPTER 1
The Running Body

Food provides the body with the energy and nutrients it needs for growth and development, to meet daily lifestyle requirements and maintain health. Food choices making up a runner's daily diet must meet all these requirements, otherwise running performance will suffer, risk of infection and injury will increase, and there may even be long-term health implications. Not only do nutrients perform different functions in the body but the type and amount of nutrients varies from food to food. Understanding what energy and nutrients do in the body and which foods are good sources of particular nutrients will help a runner to build up the best possible diet. That diet should maximize performance, both in training and races, and keep the body fit and healthy. It must also be practical and fit into the lifestyle and daily schedule of the runner – and of course it must be enjoyable!

NUTRIENTS AND THEIR MAIN FUNCTIONS

Food is made up of carbohydrate, fat, protein, vitamins, minerals and water. In some foods, particularly fruits and vegetables, a very large proportion is water; in others, such as oils and fats, the water content is minimal. The amounts and indeed the presence of the different vitamins and minerals can vary considerably between foods, too. This is one of the reasons why health professionals are constantly encouraging the general public to eat a diet containing a wide variety of different foods.

Carbohydrate and fat are the major sources of energy or fuel for the body. Protein has the unique function of providing the material for the growth and repair of the body and is also an important component of enzymes, hormones and antibodies. When the diet contains more protein than is needed it contributes to the overall energy pool of the body. If insufficient carbohydrates and fats are available to meet energy demands, protein can be used to meet the shortfall.

Vitamins and minerals are essential components of the diet. Although the majority of them are needed in very small amounts they do play vital and often very different roles in the diet. Vitamins are a diverse group of substances that are needed for the regulation of chemical processes in the body. Although not a source of energy in themselves, many of them are involved in the release of energy from food. They cannot be made in the body in sufficient amounts to meet requirements and so must be provided by the diet. Minerals are also essential nutrients, which must be supplied by the diet. Like vitamins, they fulfil many functions. They help to control the composition of body fluids, and are constituents of bones and teeth and essential components of enzymes and proteins such as haemoglobin.

ENERGY

Terms Used

It is a myth that energy is 'good' because it helps to fuel activities such as running and calories are 'bad' because they are fattening. In that case, an energy bar will help a runner but a chocolate bar will make him or her fat! Energy can be measured in calories or joules. For the scientifically minded, one calorie is the amount of heat needed to raise the temperature of 1g of water by 1°C. The calorie is a very small unit, so the Calorie, which is 1,000 times greater than the calorie, has always been used for nutritional measurements. The kilocalorie is the same as the Calorie. This avoids any confusion between calorie and Calorie (initial capital 'C') and the possibility of printing errors on food packaging. Kilocalories have been replaced by the general unit for measuring energy, the kilojoule. Although it is more scientifically correct to use 'kilojoules', 'kilocalories' still remains popular with the general public and both units are used in food labelling.

**CONVERTING CALORIES
AND JOULES**

1 kilojoule (kJ)	=	1,000 joules
1 megajoule (MJ)	=	1,000,000 joules
1 kilocalorie (kcal)	=	1,000 calories or
		1 Calorie (Cal)

To convert from one unit to another

1kcal	=	4.184kJ
1MJ	=	239kcal

Energy Needs

The actual amount of energy needed varies from individual to individual. It is primarily determined by the basal metabolic rate and level of physical activity. The basal metabolic rate (BMR) is the rate at which an individual uses energy to maintain all the bodily functions at rest. This includes the energy needed to keep breathing, keep the heart beating and the blood circulating, maintain the body temperature and the brain functioning. BMR is measured when the body is at complete rest.

In adults, the BMR is proportional to the lean body mass. As men tend to have more muscle than women, their BMR is usually higher. Older adults usually have a lower BMR than younger adults as a result of the decrease in muscle (normally) with increasing age. This of course is one of the many advantages of maintaining a high level of physical activity throughout adult life. Muscle is an active tissue and therefore has an energy requirement. This means that older runners will need to eat and enjoy more food than their more inactive friends and relatives. On average, the BMR accounts for about 75 per cent of an individual's energy needs.

The thermic effect of food (TEF) represents the increase in energy expenditure that results from digesting, absorbing, metabolizing and storing food during the day. This is the source of the myth that says that it takes more energy to digest an egg than the egg actually contains. TEF accounts for about 10 per cent of the twenty-four-hour energy expenditure. Adaptive thermogenesis (AT) is the smallest component of total energy expenditure (although it would have been a larger component hundreds of years ago before central heating was invented). It represents the energy needed in times of environmental stress such as seasonal temperature changes. The amount of energy expended being physically active is the most variable. Sitting and sleeping for most of the day will probably require no more than 100kcal whereas an average of 2,800kcal will be needed to complete a marathon distance.

Dietary Energy

All the energy needed comes from diet. Food is digested, absorbed and metabolized to release energy, which the body can then use. On a weight basis, carbohydrate, fat, protein and alcohol provide variable amounts of energy. Water on the other hand has no calorific value. 1g of protein provides 4kcal (17kJ), 1g of fat provides 9kcal (37kJ), 1g of carbohydrate provides 4kcal (17kJ) and 1g of alcohol provides 7kcal (29kJ). Almost all the weight of a food is made up of these components, plus water. Therefore foods that contain a large percentage of water, such as fruits and vegetable, will have relatively fewer calories. Fatty foods, such as butter, margarines and oils, which contain little water, will be rich in calories. In fact, most foods are a mixture of nutrients and the total energy value of a food is the sum of the energy from each of the nutrients.

Energy Storage

Carbohydrate can be stored in a limited amount in the liver and muscles as glycogen. Protein in excess of the daily requirement cannot be stored but instead may be converted in the liver into glucose and used as an immediate energy source, stored as glycogen for later use, or stored as fat. Excess fat is stored as adipose tissue. The capacity for the body to store fat is unlimited. Fat cells can just get bigger and bigger.

CARBOHYDRATES

Carbohydrates occur in the diet as simple carbohydrates or sugars and complex carbohydrates or starches. Most dietary carbohydrate is plant in origin, the exception being lactose, the sugar found in milk. The main sources of simple carbohydrates are fruits and fruit juices, milk and milk products, honey and sugar. They are identifiable by their sweet taste. Sources of complex carbohydrates include bread, rice, pasta, potatoes, breakfast cereals, pulses and sweetcorn. Runners have a much greater requirement for carbohydrate than the general public and as training increases more carbohydrate is needed. Most runners will find that they need to include some of the more sugary sources of carbohydrate as well as the more bulky starchy varieties.

After digestion, glucose from sugars and starches is absorbed into the bloodstream and transported to the liver. Some of the glucose passes directly to all the cells of the body to be used for energy. Some is converted into glycogen and stored in the liver and muscles as a readily available source of energy. Some may be converted into fatty acids and stored as adipose tissue. Carbohydrates are the main source of energy for exercising muscles, the brain and the central nervous system. The brain needs a regular and constant supply of glucose to function. When carbohydrate availability is low, through starvation, very prolonged submaximal exercise or a minimal intake of carbohydrate, ketones released from the metabolism of fat are used and they can make up to, but no more than, 50 per cent of the brain's energy requirement. Many experts see very low carbohydrate intakes as positively harmful. High levels of ketones in the blood lead to the abnormal state of ketosis, which, apart from the health aspect, can leave the dieter feeling nauseous, light-headed and suffering from rather nasty halitosis (bad breath). If the diet is low in carbohydrate a greater percentage of dietary protein is used to provide glucose so there is less protein available for growth and repair of body tissues. Carbohydrate therefore has a protein-sparing effect, which is particularly important for those involved in regular physical activity. Runners following the fashionable low-carbohydrate high-protein diets are likely to feel tired, lethargic and irritable as they become deprived of stored carbohydrate, the body's best source of energy for exercise.

DIETARY FIBRE

Fibre was originally referred to as 'roughage', its technically correct term is 'non-starch polysaccharides' (NSP), but 'dietary fibre' is the term with which most people are familiar and this remains the term that is most commonly used in food labelling. Fibre is the major component of plant cell walls. It is resistant to the action of digestive enzymes.

Most dietary fibre comes from fruit, vegetables and cereals. In wheat, maize and rice the fibre is mainly insoluble. Insoluble fibre helps to keep the bowels functioning healthily and regularly. As it absorbs water, it tends to swell in the gut, making the gut contents heavier and as a result causing them to move more quickly through the digestive system. This can help to relieve constipation and other bowel disorders. Soluble fibre occurs more frequently in oats, legumes, leafy vegetables and some fruits, particularly apples. It is thought to help reduce blood cholesterol levels and to slow down the absorption of blood glucose in some types of diabetes.

Although those in the general population are being encouraged to increase their intake of dietary fibre, runners who are already including more carbohydrate in their diet may find that their intakes of dietary fibre are already enough without adding a lot of high-fibre foods. A gut that works very quickly is not always a benefit to a runner. In some instances it can be a positive embarrassment.

GLYCAEMIC INDEX

The glycaemic index (GI) of food is a measure of that food's effect on blood glucose levels. The concept was first developed in 1981 by Dr David Jenkins, a professor of nutrition at the University of Toronto, Canada, to help patients with diabetes minimize the rise in their blood glucose after a meal. The glycaemic index classification is described as a ranking of foods based on their actual postprandial blood glucose response compared to a reference food, either glucose or white bread. It therefore reflects the speed of digestion and absorption of a carbohydrate-rich food.

However, the level of the GI of a food is not the complete picture as it is not related to portion size. For example, parsnips have a high GI but 400g of parsnips (the amount needed to provide 50g carbohydrate) would have been used for the measurement. The average portion size of parsnips is only 65g, which will contain about 8g carbohydrate. Such a small amount of carbohydrate would not have a particularly significant glycaemic effect. A more practical way of using the GI is therefore to take into consideration the usual portion size of the food.

The glycaemic load (GL) is the GI of the food multiplied by its carbohydrate content in grams. Certain foods may be more suitable for eating before running, others more suitable for refuelling after a run or race, depending on their GI or GL. The practical aspects of using the GI and its relevance to a runner's diet will be dealt with in more detail in the next chapter.

FAT

Fat is an essential nutrient and no attempt should be made to exclude it from the diet. It is an important source of energy and it supplies essential fatty acids such as linoleic acid and alpha linolenic acid, which the body cannot manufacture (hence the term 'essential'). Fat provides insulation and cushioning for the internal organs and serves as a carrier for fat-soluble vitamins (vitamin A, D, E and K) and fat-soluble antioxidants such as beta-carotene and other carotenoids. Certain essential fats are vital for the formation of hormones.

Food would taste bland without some fat in the diet as many of the flavours, smells and textures are linked to the fats in food. However, an excess amount of fat in the diet is increasingly recognized as one of the risk factors influencing the development of chronic diseases. The main concern centres on its potential role in contributing to obesity and all the associated health risks of obesity, such as heart disease. Runners who maintain a high level of physical activity still need to keep a check on their total fat intake. Enjoying a high-fat diet could mean that vital carbohydrates get pushed out of the diet. If a high carbohydrate intake is being achieved, together with a high fat intake, then even a runner will not be immune to weight increase as overall energy intake exceeds energy output.

Good and Bad Fats

Advice has always been to reduce the amount of saturated fats in the diet because they are primarily responsible for raising blood cholesterol levels. Although this still holds true, importance is now also being placed on the inclusion of other types of fat because of their positive health properties. The body uses cholesterol to

---

SOURCES OF FAT

Visible fat	Invisible fat	Invisible fat
Butter, margarine, ghee	Very lean cuts of meat	Fried food and pastry
Oils, lard, suet, dripping	Cheese	Nuts, olives, avocado pears
Hydrogenated fats and vegetable shortening (check food labels)	Whole milk – silver or gold top	Some types of cakes and biscuits
Cream	Eggs	Creamy puddings and cheesecake
Fat on meat, poultry skin	Meat products – pies, pasties, sausages, burgers, pate and salami, tinned meats	Mayonnaise, salad cream and creamy sauces
Oily fish	Chips, crisps and roast potatoes	Peanut butter
		Chocolate, toffee, fudge

---

build cell membranes as well as brain and nerve tissue. However, the body gets all it needs from cholesterol made in the liver and transported round the body in blood. Because blood is mainly composed of water, which does not mix with fat, cholesterol travels around the body attached to specific proteins or lipoproteins.

There are two types of lipoproteins: low-density lipoproteins (LDL) and high-density lipoproteins (HDL). Cholesterol is carried in the blood by low-density lipoproteins (LDL) from the liver to various tissues in the body but on the way cholesterol can also be deposited in the arteries. It is these deposits that lead to an increased risk of developing heart disease. High-density lipoproteins (HDL) carry cholesterol from the tissues back to the liver, where it is broken down. The balance of LDL and HDL cholesterol is as important as the total blood cholesterol level. Low levels of LDL and high levels of HDL cholesterol are best. Regular physical activity helps to increase the level of HDL cholesterol in the body.

Saturated Fats

A high intake of saturated fats is associated with an increase in blood cholesterol. Main sources of saturated fats are butter, cheese, meat, meat products such as sausages and hamburgers, full-fat milk and full-fat yoghurt, pies, pastries, lard, dripping, hard margarines and baking fats, coconut and palm oil.

Monounsaturated Fats

Monounsaturated fats lower LDL and so help to reduce the risk of heart disease. However, this beneficial effect may simply be the result of these fats replacing the saturated fats in the diet. Main sources of monounsaturated fats are olives, rapeseed, nuts (pistachio, almonds, hazelnuts, macadamia, cashew, pecan), peanuts, avocados and their oils.

Polyunsaturated Fats

These fats can be further divided into the omega-6 and omega-3 families. Omega-6 fats are derived from linoleic acid. Omega-3 fats, which include eicosapentaenoic acid (EPA) and docosahexaenoic acid (DHA), are produced from alpha-linolenic acid (ALA). Linoleic acid and ALA are called essential fatty acids as the body cannot make them and the diet must provide them. A diet rich in omega-6 fatty acids and low in saturated fat has been linked with a reduced risk of coronary heart disease. Advice is now also to eat more omega-3s as these are thought to have a positive impact on heart health as well as having an important role in brain and eye function. Good sources of omega-3 polyunsaturates are salmon, mackerel, herring, sardines, trout (all of which are particularly rich in EPA and DHA), eggs laid by hens consuming diets rich in omega-3 (for example, Columbus eggs), and walnuts, rapeseed, soybean, flax seed, and their oils (all particularly rich in alpha-linolenic acid). Good sources of omega-6 polyunsaturates are sunflower seeds, wheat-germ, sesame seeds, walnuts, soybean, maize and their oils and certain margarines; information is given on the tubs. Of particular interest to runners will be the anti-inflammatory properties of omega-3 fatty acids and their potential to relieve symptoms of stiffness and pain in joints (*see* Chapter 7).

Unsaturated fats can also come in different chemical structures – a bent 'cis' form or a straight 'trans' form. Most unsaturated fats come in the cis form but in the meat and milk of ruminants (cows, sheep and deer), and in products containing industrially hardened oils, some of the unsaturated fats will exist in the trans form. These are called trans fatty acids and, like saturated fats, they increase blood cholesterol levels. Some frying and baking fats (hydrogenated vegetable oils) used in biscuits, cakes, pastries, dairy products and fatty meat from beef and sheep will contain these trans fatty acids.

Dietary Recommendations

Most European guidelines now suggest that overall fat intake should be no more than 30–35 per cent of total calories, with no more than 10 per cent of calories coming from saturated fats. This means that the remaining 20–25 per cent of calories should come from mono- and polyunsaturated sources. It is also important to make a positive effort to include more omega-3 polyunsaturated fats in the diet and keep trans fats to a minimum.

CHOLESTEROL

Cholesterol is used by the body to make hormones (including the sex hormones), vitamin D, bile salts and to maintain the structure of cell membranes and it is also involved in protecting nerve fibre. Sources of cholesterol in the diet are egg yolks, offal (liver and kidney), shellfish and fish roes. Although some foods are rich in cholesterol, up to 95 per cent of the cholesterol in the body is made from dietary saturated fat. In terms of lowering blood cholesterol levels, general advice is to lower saturated fat intake rather than try to eliminate all dietary cholesterol.

PROTEIN

Proteins are an essential constituent of virtually every cell in the body, accounting for about one-fifth of the total body weight. They perform vital structural functions in the body and are constituents of muscle, connective tissue (bone, cartilage, tendons and ligaments), skin and hair. Proteins are responsible for growth and development and on a daily basis they are involved in rebuilding, repairing and maintaining vital tissues. They also have a regulatory role. Enzymes and hormones are proteinous by nature and together they regulate tissue and cell metabolism. For example, insulin is a protein that monitors blood glucose levels. Some proteins (immunoglobulins) are important in the functioning of the immune system and so help to fight off infection. Other proteins work as transporters, moving fats and minerals around the body. Oxygen is transported in the blood to all cells by the protein haemoglobin.

Although these are the primary and unique functions of protein, it can also be a source of energy. Protein cannot be stored in the body so if more is consumed than the body needs, some of the protein molecule is broken down and excreted in the urine as urea and the rest is either used for energy or converted to fat and stored.

SOURCES OF PROTEIN	
Animal sources	**Vegetable sources**
Meat	Beans, peas and lentils
Offal	Nuts and seeds
Poultry	Quorn, tofu
Fish, shellfish	Soybeans, soya milk
Eggs	Textured vegetable protein
Milk, cheese, yoghurt	Bread, potatoes, rice, pasta, cereals

Amino Acids

Amino acids are the building blocks of protein. Like carbohydrates and fats, amino acids contain carbon, hydrogen and oxygen but they also contain nitrogen and occasionally sulphur.

Amino is the chemical name for the combination of nitrogen and hydrogen in these compounds. All the proteins needed by the body can be made from just twenty different amino acids. Some amino acids can be made from others (these are called non-essential amino acids) but there are some that cannot be made by the body, which have to be supplied by the diet. These are known as essential amino acids. Cysteine and tyrosine are sometimes called semi-essential amino acids as they can only be made from the essential amino acids methionine and phenylalanine.

CLASSIFICATION OF AMINO ACIDS

Essential amino acids	Non-essential amino acids
Isoleucine	Alanine
Leucine	Arginine
Lysine	Asparagine
Methionine	Aspartic acid
Phenylalanine	Cysteine/cystine
Threonine	Glutamic acid
Tryptophan	Glutamine
Valine	Glycine
Histidine (in infants)	Proline
	Serine
	Tyrosine

Sources of Protein

Some foods contain more protein than others but actually quality is just as important as quantity. It is not just the amount of protein that matters, but also which amino acids the protein contains and whether they are present in sufficient amounts. Plant proteins tend to be low or deficient in one or more essential amino acids and therefore generally have a lower biological value than animal proteins. Animal foods (for example, meat, fish, eggs, milk and cheese) have high protein contents with high biological value. Pulses (for example, soybean, kidney beans, chickpeas, lentils and peanuts) are foods with a very high protein content with high (soya) or medium biological value. Cereals (wheat, rice, barley, maize and oats) are foods with medium protein content with medium (rice) or low biological value. Nuts (hazelnut, cashew, almond, walnut) are foods with high protein content but low biological value. Starchy roots (cassava, potato, yam and sweet potato) are low in protein and have negligible biological value. Vegetables and fruits are low in protein and are not really considered dietary sources of protein, although of course they make a valuable contribution to the diet in other ways.

Excess Protein

A high-protein diet increases the workload of the kidneys because of the extra nitrogen that must be excreted. This does not seem to be a problem in otherwise healthy people but might be problematic in physically active individuals who already have increased fluid losses through sweating.

VITAMINS AND MINERALS

Vitamins

Vitamins are complex organic substances that are needed in very small but vital amounts for many of the processes that go on in the body. Although only a few milligrams (mg) or even micrograms (µg) are needed each day they are absolutely essential for health. Most vitamins cannot be made in the body and must therefore be supplied by the diet. The exception is vitamin D, which is manufactured in the body by the action of sunlight on the skin. In addition, small amounts of niacin, a B vitamin, can be made from the amino acid tryptophan.

Vitamins perform a variety of functions in the body; some are co-factors in enzyme activity, some are antioxidants and vitamin D is a pro-hormone. A consistently poor intake of vitamins over a period of time can result in the development of a deficiency disease. Vitamin-deficiency diseases are rare in the developed world, although they still occur in some parts of the developing world. Vitamins are traditionally grouped into two categories: fat-soluble, which are stored in the body (vitamins A, D, E and K), and water-soluble, which cannot be stored in the body (vitamin C and the B complex vitamins). Any water-soluble vitamins consumed in excess of requirements are normally excreted via the kidneys in the urine.

Minerals

Minerals are inorganic substances that are needed by the body for a variety of functions. They help to build and maintain strong bones and teeth, transport oxygen around the body, regulate water and acid–base balance, activate and form essential parts of enzymes and hormones, fight infections, maintain healthy levels of haemoglobin in the blood, release energy from food, transmit nerve impulses and relax and contract muscles. Most minerals are excreted and must therefore be supplied regularly in the diet.

While deficiencies in essential nutrients can be harmful so, too, can excesses. Excessive intakes of some minerals can lead to problems ranging from nausea and vomiting to hypertension, irregular heartbeat or skin and kidney damage. An imbalance in the proportion of one mineral may cause a corresponding deficiency in another one.

How Much Is Enough?

In 1991 the UK Department of Health published guidelines for the intake of nutrients using a new term, the Reference Nutrient Intake (RNI) (Department of Health, *Dietary Reference Values for Food Energy and Nutrients for the United Kingdom*, London: HMSO, 1991 (Report on Health and Social Subjects; No. 41)). The RNI was defined as the amount of a nutrient that is enough for almost every individual, even someone who has significant needs for that nutrient. The amount is therefore considerably higher than that which most people need. You are most unlikely to become deficient in a nutrient if you consume the RNI.

VITAMINS

Vitamin A
Major food sources   Vitamin A is found in animal foods as retinol. Plant foods contain beta-carotene, the precursor of vitamin A.
Richest sources of vitamin A are fish liver oils (cod liver oil) and animal liver (lamb, calf and pig).
Good sources of vitamin A include oily fish (mackerel, herring, tuna, sardines and salmon), egg yolk, full-fat milk, butter, cheese and fortified margarine.
Good sources of beta-carotene are fruit and vegetables, especially orange ones (carrots, apricots), dark green ones (spinach, watercress and broccoli) and red ones (tomatoes and red peppers).

continued overleaf

VITAMINS *continued*

Main functions	Essential for healthy skin.
	Maintains healthy mucous membranes in the throat and nose.
	Protects against poor vision in dim light.
	Antioxidant properties.
Deficiency	Very rare in the UK.
	In developing world, deficiency is a major cause of blindness.
Requirements	Reference Nutrient Intake (RNI) for adult men is 700µg per day and for adult women 600µg per day.
Excessive intakes	Regular intakes of retinol should not exceed 7,500µg for adult women, 9,000µg for adult men and 3,300µg for pregnant women. Women who are or might become pregnant are advised by the Department of Health not to take vitamin A supplements or eat liver, as excessive amounts can be toxic and dangerous to the unborn child.

Vitamin B$_1$ (thiamin)

Major food sources	Cereal products such as breakfast cereals, bread, pasta and rice, lean pork and peas, beans and lentils.
Main functions	Release of energy from carbohydrate.
	For normal functioning of nerves, brain and muscles.
Deficiency	Very rare in the UK.
	Causes beri-beri, which affects the heart and nervous system.
Requirements	RNI for adult men is 1.0mg per day and for adult women 0.8mg per day. (Dependent on the energy content of the diet; RNI is set at 0.4mg per 1000kcal for most groups of people.)
Excessive intakes	Chronic intakes in excess of 3g per day are toxic in adults.

Vitamin B$_2$ (riboflavin)

Major food sources	Milk, egg yolks, liver, kidneys, cheese, wholemeal bread and cereals and green vegetables. Sensitive to light.
Main functions	Release of energy from carbohydrate, fat and protein.
Deficiency	Sores in the corners of the mouth.
	Severe deficiency unlikely in the UK.
Requirements	RNI for adult men is 1.3mg per day and for adult women 1.1mg per day.
Excessive intakes	Absorption of riboflavin in the intestine is limited, so toxic effects unlikely.

Niacin (nicotinic acid, nicotinamide, vitamin B$_3$)

Major food sources	Meat, poultry, fortified breakfast cereals, white flour and bread, yeast extracts.
Main functions	Release of energy from protein, fat and carbohydrate.
Deficiency	Rare.
Requirements	RNI for adult men is 17mg per day and for adult women 13mg per day.
Excessive intakes	Very high intakes in the region of 3–6g per day may cause liver damage.

VITAMINS

Vitamin B$_6$ (pyridoxine)

Major food sources	Meat, particularly beef and poultry, fish, wholemeal bread and fortified breakfast cereals.
Main functions	Needed for protein metabolism, central nervous system functioning, haemoglobin production and antibody formation.
Deficiency	Deficiency signs are rare.
Requirements	RNI for adult men is 1.4mg per day and for adult women 1.2mg per day.
Excessive intakes	High intakes have been associated with impaired function of sensory nerves. Amounts involved have varied from 50mg per day to 2 to 7g per day.

Vitamin B$_{12}$ (cyanocobalamin)

Major food sources	Found only in food of animal origin (liver, kidney, meat, oily fish, milk, cheese and eggs). Some breakfast cereals are fortified with vitamin B$_{12}$. Some vegetarian foods are fortified, for example, soya protein, soya milks, yeast extract.
Main functions	Red blood cell formation, maintenance of nervous system and protein metabolism.
Deficiency	Pernicious anaemia (blood disorder).
Requirements	RNI for adult men and women is 1.5µg per day.
Excessive intakes	Excreted in the urine and therefore not dangerous.

Folic acid (folates)

Major food sources	Liver, kidney, green leafy vegetables, wholegrain cereals, fortified breakfast cereals and breads, eggs, pulses, bananas and orange juice.
Main functions	Red and white blood cell formation in bone marrow. Essential for growth. Protection against neural tube defects (spina bifida) pre-conceptually and in early pregnancy.
Deficiency	Megaloblastic anaemia (blood disorder).
Requirements	RNI for adults is 200µg per day. Women who might become pregnant or pregnant women during the first twelve weeks of pregnancy are recommended to take an extra 400µg per day.
Excessive intakes	Dangers of toxicity are very low.

Biotin and Pantothenic acid

Major food sources	Widespread in food.
Main functions	Release of energy from fats, carbohydrates and protein.
Deficiency	Unlikely.
Requirements	None set.
Excessive intakes	No danger.

continued overleaf

VITAMINS *continued*

Vitamin C

Major food sources	Fruit and vegetables especially blackcurrants, strawberries and citrus fruit, raw peppers, tomatoes and green leafy vegetables. Potatoes because of the amount eaten.
Main functions	For healthy skin, blood vessels, gums and teeth, wound healing, iron absorption and formation of antibodies. Important antioxidant.
Deficiency	Scurvy. Mild deficiency leads to tiredness, bleeding gums, delayed wound healing and lowered resistance to infection.
Requirements	RNI for adults is 40mg per day.
Excessive intakes	Intakes at levels of twenty times RNI or more have been associated with diarrhoea and increased risk of oxalate stones in the kidney.

Vitamin D (cholecalciferol)

Major food sources	Fortified margarines and spreads, fortified breakfast cereals, oily fish, egg yolks, full-fat milk and dairy products. Main source of vitamin D is the action of UV light on the skin.
Main function	Absorption of calcium and its utilization in the body; particularly the mineralization of bones and teeth.
Deficiency	Loss of calcium from the bones, causing rickets in young children and osteomalacia particularly in women of child-bearing age.
Requirements	No dietary source needed for adults provided that skin is exposed to sunlight (RNI for adults aged 65 and over is 10µg per day).
Excessive intakes	Toxicity is rare in adults.

Vitamin E

Major food sources	Vegetable oils, seeds, nuts (especially peanuts), wheatgerm, wholemeal bread and cereals, green plants, milk and milk products and egg yolks.
Main functions	Powerful antioxidant, protecting body tissues against free-radical damage.
Deficiency	None except in very exceptional circumstances.
Requirements	No RNI set; 4µg per day for adult men and 3µg per day for adult women considered adequate.
Excessive intakes	Toxicity extremely rare.

Vitamin K

Major food sources	Dark green leafy vegetables, margarines and vegetable oils, milk and liver. Also synthesized by bacteria in the gut.
Main functions	Blood clotting.
Deficiency	Rare in adults.
Requirements	No RNI set but 1µg per kg per day is considered both safe and adequate.
Excessive intakes	Natural K vitamins seem free from toxic side-effects, even up to 100 times the safe intake. Synthetic forms may not have such a margin of safety.

MINERALS

Calcium

Major food sources   Milk, cheese and yoghurt (low-fat and full-fat), tinned sardines and pilchards (from the edible bones), dark green leafy vegetables, pulses (including baked beans), white flour and white bread (fortified) and hard water.

Main functions   Essential for strong and healthy bones and teeth.
Important in blood clotting.
Essential for nerve and muscle function.

Deficiency   Causes problems with bones, which may become brittle and break easily (osteoporosis or brittle bone disease). Good calcium intakes in childhood and adolescence are vital to help build up calcium in the bones and to protect against osteoporosis in later life.

Requirements   RNI for adult men and women is 700mg per day.
Vitamin D is essential for the absorption of calcium.

Excessive intakes   Calcium toxicity is virtually unknown. The body adapts to high intakes by reducing the amount that is absorbed.

Phosphorus

Major food sources   Present in all plant and animal foods except fats and sugars.

Main functions   Essential for the formation of bones and teeth.
Involved in many metabolic reactions.

Deficiency   Unknown.

Requirements   RNI for adult men and women is 550mg per day.

Excessive intakes   Not known in adults.

Magnesium

Major food sources   Present in most foods, particularly cereals, vegetables (especially dark green leafy ones) and fruit.

Main functions   Energy production, nerve and muscle function and bone structure.

Deficiency   Body is very efficient at regulating magnesium content, so deficiencies are rare. Usually caused by severe diarrhoea or excessive losses in the urine resulting from the use of diuretics.

Requirements   RNI for adult men is 300mg per day and for adult women 270mg per day.

Excessive intakes   No evidence that high intakes are harmful if kidney function is normal.

Sodium and chloride

Major food sources   As sodium chloride (salt). About 15–20 per cent sodium chloride naturally present in food, 15–29 per cent added in cooking or to the food once served and 60–79 per cent added during food processing or manufacture. Foods high in sodium chloride include ham, bacon, smoked fish, foods canned in brine, cheese, butter, salted nuts and biscuits, and yeast extract. Significant contributions are also made because of the amount of bread, breakfast cereal, ready meats, canned meats, savoury snacks, soups and sauces consumed on a regular basis.

continued overleaf

MINERALS *continued*

Main functions   Regulation of body water content, maintenance of acid–base balance, blood volume and blood pressure and nerve and muscle function.
Deficiency   Unlikely in normal circumstances (*see* Chapter 4)
Requirements   RNI for adult men and women 1,600mg per day for sodium and 2,500mg per day for chloride. Food Standards Agency and UK Health Departments advise to keep intakes at or below 6g salt per day.
Excessive intakes   Evidence for a direct association between salt intake and high blood pressure is now much stronger than thought a few years ago.

Potassium
Major food sources   Present in all foods except fats, oils and sugar. Particularly good sources are fruits (bananas and oranges), vegetables, potatoes, coffee, tea and cocoa.
Main functions   Regulation of fluid balance in conjunction with sodium. Potassium maintains water inside the cells (intracellular fluid) and sodium maintains water outside the cells (extracellular fluid). Appears to have a positive effect in reducing blood pressure (a reason to maintain fruit and vegetable intakes). Involved in nerve and muscle function.
Deficiency   Unlikely. Can result from severe diarrhoea and vomiting.
Requirements   RNI for adult men and women is 3,500mg per day.
Excessive intakes   Toxicity only likely to occur by supplementation.

Iron
Major food sources   Liver, lean meat (especially red meat), kidney, heart, shellfish and egg yolks. Wholegrain cereals, dried pulses and dried fruit contain iron but it is less well absorbed than iron from animal foods.
Some breakfast cereals are fortified with iron.
Vitamin C helps the absorption of iron from plant foods.
Main function   Part of haemoglobin in red blood cells which carries oxygen to all parts of the body.
Deficiency   Low haemoglobin levels cause tiredness and fatigue and ultimately iron deficiency anaemia. Iron deficiency is one of the most common nutritional deficiencies in developed and developing countries. As many as one in three women of child-bearing age in the UK is iron deficient.
Requirements   RNI for women (11–50-plus years) is 14.8mg per day. RNI for adult men is 8.7mg per day. RNI for women is higher to make up for iron losses due to monthly periods.
Excessive intakes   No risk from normal foods other than in people with rare metabolic disorders.

MINERALS

Zinc
Major food sources   Red meat, liver, shellfish (especially oysters), dairy products and eggs. Wholegrain cereals, bread and pulses contain zinc but it is less well absorbed.

Main functions   Part of many enzymes needed for a variety of body functions, involved in energy production, aiding wound healing, in development of the body's immune system (antioxidant function) and in insulin production.

Deficiency   Insufficient zinc can slow growth and development. It also delays wound healing and may impair immune function.

Requirements   RNI for adult men is 9.5mg per day and for adult women 7.0mg per day.

Excessive intakes   Acute ingestion of 2g of zinc produces nausea and vomiting. Long-term intakes of 50mg per day interfere with copper metabolism.

Copper
Major food sources   Present in trace quantities in many foods.

Main functions   Part of many enzyme systems, particularly those involved in metabolism and antioxidant function.

Deficiency   May have a role in the development of heart disease but more research is needed.

Requirement   RNI for adult men and women is 1.2mg per day.

Excessive intakes   High intakes are toxic but these only occur in abnormal circumstances such as contaminated water.

Selenium
Major food sources   Wholegrain cereals, meat, fish and shellfish, milk and egg yolks and Brazil nuts.
Selenium content of food is dependent on the amount in the soil.

Main function   Powerful antioxidant (protects cell membranes).

Deficiency   No clinical condition associated with a dietary deficiency but possible link with the development of heart disease.

Requirements   RNI for adult men is 75µg per day and for adult women 60µg per day.

Excessive intakes   High levels (in excess of 1mg) are known to be toxic and an upper limit of 6µg per kg per day for adults has been set.

Fluoride
Major food sources   Drinking water with a high natural or added fluoride level, fluoride toothpaste, fish and tea.

Main function   Bone and tooth mineralization and helping in the prevention of tooth decay.

Deficiency   Increased susceptibility to tooth decay and lack of bone strength.

Requirements   No RNI set.

Excessive intakes   Causes mottling of teeth.

continued overleaf

MINERALS *continued*

Iodine

Major food sources	Only natural rich source is seafood. Other sources are milk and milk products and iodized salt.
Main function	Functioning of the thyroid and formation of thyroid hormones.
Deficiency	Resulting deficiency of thyroid hormone leads to a low metabolic rate and lethargy.
Requirements	RNI for adult men and women is 140µg per day.
Excessive intakes	Not usually a problem.

Manganese

Major food sources	Tea.
Main function	Component of many enzymes.
Deficiency	Unobserved except in experimental studies.
Requirements	No RNI set but safe intakes are believed to lie above 1.4mg per day for adults.
Excessive intakes	One of the least toxic elements. Excess intakes are quickly excreted.

Chromium

Major food sources	Meat, wholegrain cereals, legumes, nuts and brewer's yeast.
Main function	Formation of insulin and lipoprotein metabolism.
Deficiency	Unlikely on a normal mixed diet.
Requirements	No RNI set but safe intakes are believed to lie above 25µg per day for adults.

Molybdenum

Major food sources	Trace amounts found in many foods.
Main function	Enzyme function.
Deficiency	Reported on very low intakes (25µg per day); typical UK diet provides a mean of 128µg per day.
Requirements	No RNI set but safe intakes are believed to lie between 50 and 400µg per day.

Vitamin and Mineral Supplements

Vitamin and mineral supplements are generally unnecessary. Most people manage to meet their individual requirements by eating a diet that supplies enough energy to match requirements, and contains a fairly wide variety of foods. Users of supplements can be divided into three groups: those who should be taking them, those who may need to take them as a result of a poor diet or an increased requirement for a nutrient, and those who take them but probably do not need to. This last group are really just using them as an insurance policy to top up the diet, which, in the vast majority of cases, will not need to be topped up. If supplements are used they should be taken regularly and only in the recommended daily dosage.

ANTIOXIDANT NUTRIENTS

The term 'antioxidant nutrients' covers a group of vitamins, minerals and plant substances variously called phytochemicals, bioactive compounds or phytoprotectants, which act as a defence against certain diseases. When oxygen is used in chemical reactions in the body it produces potentially harmful chemicals as by-products. These 'free radicals' are unstable molecules that have part of their structure missing. As they try to replace the missing bit by 'stealing' from other molecules, they can cause damage to tissues in the body, which may ultimately cause heart disease and some cancers. The body has powerful defence mechanisms to prevent this damage occurring but these can be impaired by environmental pollutants such as cigarette smoke, car fumes and excessive exposure to sunlight. Antioxidants can neutralize free radicals by giving up the missing part to the free radical without becoming unstable themselves.

Antioxidant vitamins include vitamin A and its precursor beta-carotene and other carotenoids, vitamin C and vitamin E. Minerals with antioxidant properties include zinc, iron, copper and selenium. Phytochemicals found particularly in fruit and vegetables also act as antioxidants and include lycopene (tomatoes), saponins (onions), allicin (garlic) and indoles (broccoli, cabbage and Brussels sprouts). The advice to eat at least five portions of fruit and vegetables every day relates to the powerful antioxidant properties of such foods. There is strong evidence that including more fruit and vegetables in the daily diet could reduce the incidence of many of the major killer diseases. Indeed, some countries, most notably Australia, are recommending as many as seven or more portions of fruit and vegetables a day.

Antioxidants are not just involved in protecting the body against major diseases, they also play a part in preventing minor infections such as colds, sore throats, chest infections and so on. Runners who get more than their fair share of infections, resulting in frequent disruption to their training programme, should keep a close eye on how many portions of fruit and vegetables they have on a regular daily basis.

HOW ALCOHOL AFFECTS THE BODY

Stimulates the heart to beat faster.

Widens blood vessels (flushing and warm sensation).

Diverts blood to the skin causing loss of body heat.

Stimulates gastric juices.

Causes co-ordination and balance problems.

Slows reaction times.

Affects intellectual and sexual performance.

Regular drinking can seriously damage the liver and heart.

Brutal facts about alcohol

Alcoholic drinks are concentrated sources of calories and anyone trying to lose weight should avoid or at least restrict consumption.

Alcoholic drinks contain negligible amounts of essential nutrients such as vitamins and minerals. Excessive intake actually impairs the absorption of vitamins B_1, folic acid, B_{12} and C.

Hangovers are caused by the dehydrating effect of alcohol acting as a diuretic, taking fluid from the body and increasing urine output. The non-alcoholic congeners, which give flavour, smell and colour (where appropriate) to a drink, also contribute to the symptoms of a hangover.

Women break down alcohol more slowly than men so the intoxicating effects for the same amount of alcohol are apparent for longer.

ALCOHOL

Alcohol (ethanol) is produced when sugars are fermented by yeasts. During fermentation the yeasts grow by feeding on the sugars and producing alcohol and carbon dioxide as by-products. Fermentation has been used for thousands of years to produce alcoholic drinks and foods such as bread. Grapes and apples are used to make wines and cider, while cereals such as barley and rye form the basis for beers and spirits. After ingestion, some alcohol is quickly absorbed from the stomach, the remainder being absorbed from the small intestine. After absorption, blood-alcohol levels rise and as the 'alcoholic blood' circulates around the body it acts first as a stimulant and then, in some cases, as a depressant. Eventually, it is metabolized in the liver at a rate of about one unit or 10ml alcohol per hour, after which the breakdown products can be used as a source of energy or converted into fat and stored. Alcohol as a source of energy for running is limited.

THE WHOLE DIET APPROACH

Enjoying a diet that contains a wide variety of different foods can ensure that daily requirements for all the essential nutrients are met. Neither a monotonous diet including the same limited choice of foods nor a diet that is consistently low in overall food intake will achieve this. These are not the ways to maximize running performance or keep the running body fit and healthy. Putting foods into groups according to the main nutrients they supply makes it easier to choose wisely but enjoyably. Those who eat the correct proportions of foods from the main food groups every day, and vary the choices within each group, will be eating well and therefore probably performing better. The actual amount eaten will of course depend on individual energy requirements.

THE FIVE MAIN FOOD GROUPS

**Breads, other cereals
and starchy carbohydrates**

Foods   Bread, potatoes, pasta and noodles, rice, breakfast cereals, oats, maize, millet and cornmeal, yams and plantains. Beans, peas and lentils are also included in this group.

Function   Provide carbohydrate, calcium, iron, B vitamins and dietary fibre.

Fruit and vegetables

Foods   Fresh, frozen, dried and canned fruit and vegetables, salad vegetables and fruit juice.

Function   Provide vitamin C, carotenes, folates, carbohydrate and dietary fibre.

Milk and dairy products

Foods   Milk, cheese, yoghurt and fromage frais (but not butter, eggs or cream).

Function   Provide protein, calcium, vitamin B_{12}, vitamins A and D (lower-fat versions contain less of these fat-soluble vitamins).

Meat, fish and alternatives

Foods   Meat, poultry, fish, eggs, nuts, beans, peas and lentils.

Function   Provide protein, iron, B vitamins, zinc and magnesium. Beans, peas and lentils also provide dietary fibre.

**Foods containing fat and
foods containing sugar**

Foods   Margarine, butter and other spreading fats (including low-fat spreads), cooking oils, oil-based salad dressings, mayonnaise, cream, chocolate, crisps, biscuits, pastries, cakes, puddings, ice cream, rich sauces and gravies. Soft drinks, sweets, jam, honey, marmalade, biscuits, pastries, cakes, puddings, ice cream.

Function   Foods containing fat provide fat, essential fatty acids, some vitamins. Foods containing sugar provide carbohydrate; some minerals and vitamins and fat in some products (but not others).

The general advice relating to nutrition for long-term health is of course relevant to a marathon runner, and the diet that the general public is encouraged to follow is broadly suitable for a runner training for a marathon. However, the runner needs to incorporate some significant adaptations. Runners need to follow a high-carbohydrate diet and may therefore need to include more sugary sources as well as the starchier ones. Getting all the carbohydrate from high-fibre foods can make a diet bulky and could cause unwanted gastrointestinal side-effects. Given the amount of carbohydrate that will be consumed, particularly as mileage increases, dietary recommendations for dietary fibre will almost certainly be met without the inclusion of high-fibre breads and cereals. However, runners who prefer these foods should not exclude them from the diet unless they do cause gastrointestinal problems (*see* Chapter 7).

The advice to avoid high intakes of fat, to ensure vitamin and mineral intakes are optimum, and to keep to a sensible intake of alcohol is just as important for the marathon runner as for the general public. However, advice to cut back salt or sodium intake may not be appropriate for all runners, as it may increase the risk of developing hyponatraemia (*see* Chapter 3).

SIGNIFICANT FACTS ABOUT THE HUMAN BODY

The smallest cell in the body is the red blood cell, which is only seven-thousandths of a millimetre across. Its only function is to carry oxygen. Red blood cells live for four months, but travel about 1,500km (935 miles) around the body during that time.

There are 639 muscles in the human body. The longest is the gluteus maximus (large buttock muscle) and the shortest is the stapedius (in the middle ear).

The heart weighs less than half a kilogram and will beat about 3,000 million times and pump 400 million litres of blood during a lifetime. This equals the amount of petrol needed to fill 10 million cars.

There are 100,000km (62,500 miles) of blood vessels in the body, equivalent to twice the distance around the world.

The nervous system sends messages as fast as 300km (around 185 miles) per hour.

From *The Human Atlas* by Mark Crocker (Oxford University Press)

FOOD AS FUEL

So, how does the body use the energy and nutrients in food to good effect when running? A basic understanding of digestion and absorption will help you appreciate how food on the plate becomes fuel for the muscles.

Digestion

In the Mouth

Chewing in the mouth immediately starts the breakdown of food. Saliva secreted from glands in the mouth mixes with the food, making swallowing easier. It also contains an enzyme (ptyalin), which initiates carbohydrate digestion. Once it has been swallowed, the food passes down the oesophagus to the stomach in about three seconds.

In the Stomach

Gastric juices secreted from the stomach lining contain pepsin, an enzyme that begins the digestion of proteins, hydrochloric acid, which destroys most of the bacteria present in food and provides the acid conditions for pepsin to work effectively, and intrinsic factor, which is needed for absorption of vitamin B_{12} later. Mechanical breakdown continues as the stomach muscle contracts and relaxes. The stomach acts as a reservoir and food remains here for one to four hours, after which the semi-liquid is released in small amounts from the stomach into the small intestine. Foods rich in carbohydrate pass into the small intestine faster than high-fat foods. Liquids generally pass through more quickly than solid food. Stress and nerves before a race can reduce the rate of gastric emptying. Apart from absorption of water and alcohol, very little else is absorbed from the stomach.

In the Small Intestine

The small intestine is actually the longest part of the gastrointestinal tract, being about 3m long, whereas the large intestine is only 1m long. However, the large intestine has a diameter of 6cm whereas the small intestine is much narrower, at only 2–4cm. The small intestine consists of three distinct parts: the duodenum, jejunum and ileum. Bile, which is produced in the liver and stored in the gall bladder, breaks down fat into tiny droplets for digestion. Juices produced in the pancreas neutralize the acid stomach contents and continue the breakdown of fats into fatty acids, proteins into peptides and amino acids, and starch into maltose. Finally, juices produced in the actual wall of the small intestine complete the breakdown of carbohydrates into the simplest sugars – glucose, fructose and galactose. The final phase of digestion therefore occurs actually in the intestinal wall.

In the Large Intestine

The large intestine is made up of the colon, rectum and anus. Water that was used in digestion is reabsorbed. Very little food passes through the system completely undigested. This is because bacteria in the colon break down fibre residues such as cellulose by fermentation to produce gases and fatty acids. As water is removed, the faeces become dried and more solid as they pass along the rectum before being expelled from the anus. It normally takes between one and three days for food to complete the whole process from mouth to anus. The number of times people defecate is very variable. Anything from three times a day to once every three days is considered normal.

Absorption

Small amounts of water, alcohol, sugars, soluble minerals like salt and the soluble C and B vitamins can pass through the stomach lining into the bloodstream. However, most of the absorption of nutrients takes place through the walls of the small intestine. The final products of digestion that are absorbed are peptides and amino acids from proteins, fatty acids from fats, and glucose, fructose and galactose from carbohydrates.

FATE OF MAJOR NUTRIENTS IN THE BODY

Carbohydrates
1. Transported to all cells; energy provision.
2. Converted into glycogen; stored in the liver and skeletal muscles; readily available energy source.
3. Converted into fatty acids; stored as body fat; potential energy source.

Fats
Rebuilt into triglycerides; carried by lymphatic system to blood; stored as body fat; triglycerides stored in muscles.

Proteins
Amino acids carried to the liver; join the amino acid pool in the circulation; converted into other amino acids; oxidized for energy often after conversion into glucose or converted and stored as fat.

MUSCLE FIBRES

Two main types of muscle fibre can be classified on the basis of their speed of contraction and their metabolic characteristics: Type I, or slow-twitch fibres, and Type II, or fast-twitch fibres. Although it is convenient to classify them in this way, Type II fibres can be further sub-divided into Type IIa and Type IIb. The relative proportion of each fibre type varies in the same muscle of different people and in different muscles within the same person. Muscle fibres are adaptable and, although the distribution of fibre types is genetically determined, their characteristics can be changed dramatically by an appropriate training programme.

Non-elite runners have a wide spread of muscle-fibre types. During distance running, Type I fibres are recruited and only in the later stages of long runs, when Type I fibres fatigue, will Type II fibres be used. Most of the time only a small number of muscles are needed to take care of all the day-to-day

CHARACTERISTICS OF MUSCLE-FIBRE TYPES

Type I: slow-twitch or slow-oxidative fibres have the following characteristics:

- contract and relax slowly (but still many times a second);
- resistant to fatigue;
- better adapted to low-intensity, long-duration endurance work;
- high capacity for aerobic respiration;
- greater ability to utilize oxygen;
- elite marathon runners will have a high proportion of Type I fibres as they need to maintain sub-maximal effort over a prolonged period of time.

Type IIa: fast-twitch or fast-oxidative fibres have the following characteristics:

- can work both aerobically and anaerobically (with or without oxygen);
- less aerobic capacity than slow-twitch fibres;
- more aerobic capacity than fast-glycolytic fibres;
- moderate fatigue resistance;
- fibres seem to change their characteristics in response to training loads or stresses.

Type IIb: fast-twitch or fast-glycolytic fibres have the following characteristics:

- contract twice as fast as slow-twitch fibres;
- fatigue quickly;
- important for anaerobic exercise;
- elite sprinters will have a high proportion of Type IIb fibres.

pavement walking – muscles not used to this activity can become sore. This is known as 'delayed onset muscle soreness' (DOMS). These 'new' muscles need time to recover, which explains the importance of rest days and the inclusion of other forms of exercise in a well-planned training programme. Runners can achieve greater strength and fitness by allowing sufficient recovery time and making sure that muscles are not over-used.

ENERGY SYSTEMS

The rate at which energy is needed to keep up the required exercise intensity will dictate which energy system is used. Muscle fibres can use all systems but the dominance of one system over another gives the fibre its own energy characteristics. The end point of each system is the production of a highly energy-rich phosphate compound called adenosine triphosphate, or ATP. ATP is present in all living cells and when it is broken down chemical energy is released. Without ATP, muscles cannot contract and no work can be accomplished. Unfortunately, muscle only contains enough ATP to exercise maximally for one second.

To maintain muscle contractions and the ability to carry on exercising, ATP must be continually resynthesized from adenosine diphosphate (ADP). The more intense the level of exercise, the more rapidly this resynthesis must take place. Distance running on the other hand needs ATP to be provided at a consistent rate over a relatively long period of time. This is why there are three energy systems, so that the body can cope with the various demands placed on exercising muscles.

activities. However, when new activities are introduced – for example, joining a gym, running for the first time, playing squash instead of tennis, or hill-walking instead of flat

Phosphocreatine System

This system uses another energy-rich compound, phosphocreatine (PC), which breaks down in a similar way to ATP to release energy very rapidly. Rather than use this energy directly for muscle contraction, the body uses it to resynthesize ATP. Creatine phosphate is also limited in the muscle and probably only supplies enough energy for a further 5–10 seconds. The ATP-CP energy system, which does not need oxygen, is a characteristic of the fast-twitch fibres (Type IIa and Type IIb). Energy can be produced very quickly but only for 8–10 seconds. Throwing, powerlifting, jumping and 20-metre sprinting are activities that will rely heavily on this energy system.

Glycolysis

Muscle glycogen is the main source of fuel for this system. ATP is produced rapidly but not as rapidly as in the ATP-CP system. It kicks in after 8–10 seconds of intense exercise, when the ATP-CP system starts to flag. Glycolysis occurs in both the presence and absence of oxygen. During exercise of a lower intensity, glycolysis can be sustained by oxygen obtained by normal respiration. As the intensity level increases, the rate of glycolysis increases to meet the demand for ATP. Eventually, the requirement for ATP can no longer be met by aerobic glycolysis and proportionally more anaerobic glycolysis is needed. This energy system is capable of producing energy at a fairly rapid rate but it cannot produce energy for prolonged periods. It is the preferred energy system in 400- or 800-metre sprints, weight-training sessions and any all-out 90-second activity.

Aerobic Glycolysis (Aerobic Energy System)

This system requires oxygen and uses carbohydrate and fat as the primary sources of fuel for ATP production. The main sources of carbohydrate are the limited stores of muscle and liver glycogen. The main sources of fat are the small amounts of fat stored in the muscles as well as the stores of fat under the skin and the much larger (sometimes too large) deposits deeper in the body. Even in the leanest of runners the stores of adipose tissue represent a vast potential of energy. Although protein is not usually used as a source of energy, it may be used towards the end of a marathon as glycogen stores become depleted. Aerobic glycolysis has the ability to produce more ATP than the other systems but at a slower rate. The actual speed depends on the type of fuel used.

Hitting the Wall

More energy can be produced by metabolizing carbohydrate than fat for a given amount of oxygen, making it a more efficient fuel. However, its poor storage capacity can have a limiting effect on performance. Rate of glycolysis and therefore glucose oxidation decreases as glycogen stores become depleted. At this stage a runner starts to slow down as the rate of ATP production slows and power output decreases. By slowing down, fatty acid oxidation can be used to meet a greater proportion of the energy demand. This is what runners call 'hitting the wall' (and cyclists call 'bonking').

ENERGY STORES IN THE BODY

	Male	Female
Liver glycogen	90g	70g
Muscle glycogen	400g	300g
Intramuscular fat	500g	500g
Adipose tissue	7–10kg	12–20kg

Normal body stores of fat and carbohydrate in a typical 70kg male athlete and a typical 60kg female athlete.

MAXIMAL OXYGEN CONSUMPTION

There is a level of work beyond which the oxygen uptake of a runner ceases to increase, even with additional effort. This is known as the maximal aerobic capacity of a runner, or VO_2max. It is the maximum volume of oxygen that can be used in one minute during exercise. Those runners with muscles that use oxygen at a higher rate can make ATP at a faster rate. They can therefore exercise more intensely during endurance events, in other words, they can run faster. VO_2max is directly related to the maximum cardiac output (the maximum amount of blood pumped by the heart per minute), the ability to get oxygen to the muscles, and the ability of muscles to extract and use oxygen from the blood. In turn, this is related to the percentage of slow-twitch muscles. The VO_2max is largely genetically determined, mainly because muscle-fibre composition is genetically determined. However, estimates suggest that it can be improved by 10 to 20 per cent with training. Males generally have a higher VO_2max than females because they have less body fat, higher levels of haemoglobin in the blood, more muscle and a larger heart. VO_2max falls with age, as does maximal heart rate.

Although there is a reasonable relationship between VO_2max and marathon running speed, it is not the only factor that makes an elite marathon runner. Faster runners are also able to run at a higher fraction of their VO_2max over any given distance. With training, runners can increase their ability to use a larger fraction of their VO_2max, and for longer, even though their VO_2max remains the same.

RUNNING ECONOMY

Running style is an individual characteristic that can be modified by training to be more economical so it becomes possible to run at a lower VO_2max over given distances. This does not mean that excessive mileage will continue to be beneficial but certainly elite distance runners use 5 to 10 per cent less oxygen than non-elite runners. The oxygen cost of running at a constant speed increases over time – in other words, the further the distance covered, the more running economy falls. This is in part due to the gradual change in fuel source, from carbohydrate to fat, but also because the fatigued runner becomes less well-coordinated. Muscle recruitment patterns change as a runner tires, leading to a fall in running efficiency. Stride length and frequency can have a bearing on running economy too. A well-planned training programme and a high-carbohydrate diet that maintains muscle glycogen stores are the best ways to train the body to run more economically.

WHICH ENERGY SOURCE?

Approximately two-thirds of the energy requirements at rest are derived from fat metabolism and one third from carbohydrate metabolism. During exercise, the relative amounts of fat and carbohydrate that are used depend on intensity, duration and frequency of training, daily diet (which influences fuel stores) and fitness level.

Fuel for running can be supplied by fat, carbohydrate and protein, either directly from the diet or from body stores. Alcohol is an additional source of fuel but of little benefit to a runner. Which fuel is utilized depends on the body's ability to store the nutrient, the energy cost of converting it into a suitable form for storage and the specific fuel requirements of certain tissues.

Alcohol takes the highest priority because there is nowhere to store it in the body and the energy cost of converting alcohol to fat is

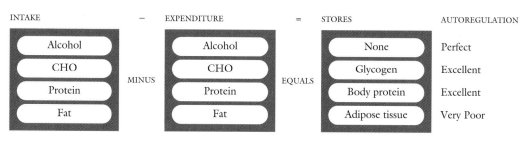

INTAKE		EXPENDITURE		STORES	AUTOREGULATION
Alcohol		Alcohol		None	Perfect
CHO	MINUS	CHO	EQUALS	Glycogen	Excellent
Protein		Protein		Body protein	Excellent
Fat		Fat		Adipose tissue	Very Poor

The hierarchy for fuel utilization.

high. Similarly, there is no storage pool for protein. The body has a limited capacity to store carbohydrate as glycogen and conversion to fat is also costly. It is necessary at all times for the body to have enough glycogen to keep blood-glucose levels steady, yet storage is limited. As a result there has to be a very tight autoregulation between the intake and oxidation of carbohydrate. In other words, when more carbohydrate is eaten, more is oxidized and vice versa. On the other hand, there is virtually no autoregulation of fat balance. When extra fat is eaten, fat oxidation hardly changes at all, partly because storage fat is virtually unlimited. There has therefore been no need to evolve an accurate method for regulating fat balance.

Protein is not a major energy source during exercise. This is because supplies must be preserved so that it can fulfil its unique function of growth and repair. However, in prolonged distance running, where carbohydrate stores become depleted, protein can make a useful contribution to total energy production. Even so, its contribution is only 3 to 6 per cent of the total energy requirement.

Fatty acids cannot be utilized in high-intensity exercise but they are vital in distance running as their supply is virtually limitless. If fat were the only fuel used to run a marathon, only 300g of fat would be needed. Even the leanest of runners would have enough. However, it is not an ideal fuel. Not only does fat produce less ATP per litre of oxygen than carbohydrate, but it is also produced at a slower rate. Somewhere between 10 and 50 per cent of the energy needed to run a marathon comes from the metabolism of fat. With training, muscles develop a greater ability to metabolize fat and this has a sparing effect on the limited carbohydrate stores.

Muscle glycogen is the body's immediate energy source. For a given volume of oxygen, carbohydrate produces 12 per cent more energy than fat. If carbohydrate were the only fuel to be used to provide energy, a marathon runner would need 700g. This is more than the amount normally stored in the body. The rapidity with which glycogen stores are used depends mainly on exercise intensity – increasing the intensity causes more glycogen to be used. As muscle glycogen stores become depleted, liver glycogen is metabolized and glucose from the liver is carried via the blood to the exercising muscles. Liver stores are also limited and eventually this source of glucose runs out, too. Endurance training increases the capacity of muscles to store glycogen. Trained runners have 20 to 50 per cent more muscle glycogen than untrained people. A trained endurance runner will therefore be more effective at carbohydrate loading prior to a marathon than a less well-trained runner. Ingestion of carbohydrate in the form of drinks and gels during long training runs and marathons can be beneficial, particularly to the non-elite runner.

Initially, energy is provided by the anaerobic pathway because it takes time for the heart and circulation to transport oxygen to the muscles and for the muscles then to utilize it. This is why the warm-up is so important. As the body settles into running, the aerobic pathway begins to kick in. The body does not switch from one system to another. Instead, the systems are used together with one pathway gradually being phased in and the other gradually phased out. Marathon running is classified as an aerobic exercise but even a marathon runner will use the anaerobic system more in certain situations, including at the start, when tackling a hilly course or attempting a sprint finish.

FLUID BALANCE

Total body water is kept at a constant level on a long-term basis although there are obviously fluctuations during the day. Excess fluid is excreted by the kidneys in response to a fall in plasma osmolality and sodium concentration. Osmosis is the movement of water from a more dilute solution to a more concentrated one across a semi-permeable membrane, in other words, one that allows water across but not necessarily the substances that are dissolved in the water. Osmolality is a measure of the osmotic pressure (OP) that a fluid exerts across the membrane and is therefore a measure of the concentration or dilution of a particular solution. This is generally determined by the number of particles dissolved or in the solution. Two solutions that exert the same OP are called isotonic. If the two solutions are not the same, the one with a higher OP is called hypertonic and the other hypotonic. Osmolality plays a part in the way fluids move from one compartment to another, for example, across the gut wall into the circulating blood. This obviously has a huge relevance

when considering the type of fluid to be drunk during training and races (*see* Chapter 3).

Body Temperature

The body temperature must be maintained between narrow limits. Although a range of skin temperatures can be tolerated, the core temperature (in other words, the temperature of the part of the body that contains the brain, heart, lungs and kidneys) must be maintained at around 37°C. When food is converted into work much of the available energy is lost as heat in the process. During exercise, when the demand for energy is increased, the rate of heat generated by the working muscles rises correspondingly. At rest, the rate of heat production is about 1kcal per minute but elite runners can produce heat at a rate of 20kcal per minute throughout a two- or three-hour training session or race. Increased heat production soon overloads the body's usual mechanisms for removing heat from the body, namely conduction, convection and radiation. As these become less effective, heat loss is achieved by the evaporation of sweat from the skin surface.

The body has several million sweat glands, which can open up, leading to a secretion of sweat on to the skin surface. As the sweat evaporates from the skin the body cools down. Water is lost first from the blood, then from the fluid that bathes the cells (extracellular fluid) and eventually from water inside the cells (intercellular fluid). Evaporation of 1 litre of water from the skin removes 590kcal of heat from the body. High rates of sweat loss are therefore essential during prolonged intense exercise if the rise in body temperature is to be limited and the loss of performance capacity that would otherwise occur is to be minimized. Evaporation of sweat can account for 80 per cent of heat loss during exercise in warm, humid conditions, rising to as much as

98 per cent in hot, dry conditions. However, loss of large amounts of sweat can lead to dehydration and electrolyte losses and this can also have a negative impact on performance.

The rate of sweating is highly variable and individual losses exceeding 2 litres an hour can occur in certain circumstances. In cool conditions, sweating usually begins about seven minutes after exercise has started.

CONSEQUENCES OF DEHYDRATION

Increase in cardiovascular strain.
Increase in thermal stress.
Increase in glycogen utilization.
Increase in muscle lactate production.
Increase in perceived rate of exertion.
Overall decrease in performance.

Dehydration

If fluid is lost faster than it is ingested and absorbed, the body gradually becomes dehydrated. As a result, not only is performance impaired, but health is also put at risk. The function of the plasma volume (fluid part of the blood) is to take oxygen and fuel to the working muscles, remove waste products and carry heat to the skin for removal. If sweat losses are not replaced by fluid intakes, the plasma volume drops. As a result, the heart rate increases to maintain cardiac output (the amount of blood pumped out with each heartbeat). Blood flow to the exercising muscles takes priority so that oxygen and fuel can continue to be supplied to them. Blood flow to the skin is consequently reduced, sweat rate falls and body temperature rises. Performance suffers as a result but, more importantly, the situation can present a health risk leading to heat exhaustion or even heat stroke (*see* Chapter 6).

RECOVERY

The body must return to normal physiological balance after a hard training session before another training session can be undertaken. Ancient man had to be able to respond to the next challenge whether it was to flee from an imminent danger or to hunt and gather his next

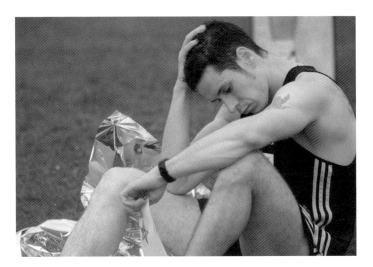

An exhausted runner recovers after completing the course. (EMPICS)

**THE RECOVERY PROCESS –
WHAT HAPPENS?**

Return of body temperature to normal.
Restoration of fluid and electrolyte balance.
Restocking of fuel stores.
Repair of damaged tissues.
Start of the adaptation process.
Risk of illness or infection minimized.
Psychological recovery so there is a desire
to go out and train again.

---

meal. This is perhaps why the recovery process begins so soon after exercise stops. Nature seems to know best in another area, too. Unfamiliar exercise, such as running uphill rather than on the flat, can lead to delayed onset muscle soreness (DOMS). This is not a pleasant sensation and runners may not feel inclined to run for a day or two, thereby allowing time for repair to take place and preventing further damage.

Restoring Fluid and Nutrient Balance

Body temperature can be reduced by beginning the recovery process in a cool room if this is possible. Drinking sufficient cool drinks and maintaining fluid intake for some hours after the training run will also bring the temperature down and replace fluid and electrolytes lost through sweating. Restoring fluid balance also

---

**KEY FACTORS INVOLVED IN
GLYCOGEN RESYNTHESIS**

Amount of carbohydrate.
Timing of carbohydrate ingestion.
Type of carbohydrate.
Type and amount of other macronutrients
present.

---

influences the physiological environment for the overall recovery process to take place. Muscle glycogen stores will have been depleted and need to be restored. Glycogen synthase, the enzyme involved in glycogen resynthesis, becomes activated immediately after prolonged exercise. Carrier proteins responsible for the uptake of blood glucose by the muscles are also increased and remain elevated for some time after exercise.

An intake of 1–1.2g carbohydrate per kg body weight immediately after the training run and at two-hourly intervals until the next meal is recommended to maximize glycogen resynthesis. However, there is no evidence that more than 100g in a two-hour period is any more beneficial. Intake of carbohydrate, particularly in the form of high-glycaemic foods and fluids, causes an increase in insulin production, which in turn maintains the elevated level of carrier proteins. Carbohydrate intake is also important if there is localized tissue damage. Including a small amount of protein with the carbohydrate may be more effective in restoring muscle glycogen stores than the same amount of carbohydrate alone. Recent research has suggested another possible advantage of consuming protein in the recovery phase. It may promote muscle protein synthesis and reduce post-exercise muscle protein breakdown. This would encourage rapid tissue repair and help prevent muscle soreness developing as weekly mileage increases.

Sleep

Sleep is a very important part of the recovery process; indeed, research has shown that those whose lifestyle includes a high level of physical activity sleep more deeply and for longer than those who are less active. Runners should not be surprised that they find they need more sleep – another example of Mother Nature knowing best.

During sleep all but the essential functions stop and instead physiological repair and growth take place, peaking during periods of deep sleep. Runners who do not get enough sleep may find that cardiovascular performance, reaction times and ability to reason logically and make decisions effectively (cognitive ability) dip.

There are several practical ways to ensure quality sleep. Going to bed at the same time each night helps the body to feel drowsy naturally. As a result there should be less difficulty getting to sleep than if bedtime is variable. An optimal environment for sleep is one that is quiet, dark, cool (ideally 18°C/65°F) and comfortable. A big bed is better than a narrow one as there can be forty to sixty position changes in the night and having enough room to turn over is obviously important.

THE EFFECTS OF TRAINING

Immune Function

Positive changes to the immune system take place during every session of moderate physical activity. Surveys have shown that those who walk briskly for thirty to forty-five minutes five times a week take fewer days off sick through an upper respiratory tract infection (URTI) than inactive individuals. However, a heavy training schedule can suppress the immune system and lead to a greater risk of an URTI. The risk can be further increased if a runner is not sleeping well, feels stressed, has a poor diet or if there is unnecessary or rapid weight loss. A runner is particularly vulnerable after a hard training session lasting more than ninety minutes. Many components of the immune system are suppressed, relating in part to the elevation of stress hormones, which are secreted in high doses during and after hard exercise, and the increased production of free

radicals. This impaired immunity can last between three and seventy-two hours, during which time viruses and bacteria can invade the body more easily. The risk of infection after a marathon is two to six times higher than normal, depending on the time of year.

Regular, but not excessive (and unnecessary) training does lead to adaptations that help to protect the body against oxidative stress associated with an increased production of free radicals. Runners need to ensure that their diet provides adequate energy to meet requirements and that it is rich in antioxidant nutrients. Studies have shown that using a sports drink before, during and after training can minimize any rise in the stress hormones cortisol, catecholamines and growth hormone. A rise in these hormones has a negative effect on immunity. The risk of picking up an infection can therefore be reduced by use of a suitable sports drink.

Sports Anaemia

When a runner follows a hard training programme, one of the responses to aerobic exercise is an increase in plasma volume. Although the number of red blood cells and therefore the amount of haemoglobin remains the same, it appears to be less because it is diluted by the increased plasma volume. The concentration of haemoglobin appears lower but the ability to carry oxygen around the body is not reduced. This is often called 'sports anaemia', an unfortunate misnomer as it implies a lack of iron in the diet or the need for an iron supplement, which is not the case.

BODY COMPOSITION

Excess body fat can reduce the speed and endurance of a marathon runner. If two runners weighing the same but with a different body composition run with each other, the one with more muscle and less body fat will have a distinct performance advantage. Body fat content tends to fall as training volume increases and for the runner carrying excessive amounts of body fat this will have a beneficial effect on performance as less 'dead weight' needs to be carried over the distance. A non-elite runner will tend to have up to twice as much body fat as an elite runner. However, it is important to remember that having too little body fat is not only counterproductive to performance but also dangerous to general health and fitness.

Body Fat

The body contains two main types of fat: essential fat and storage fat. Essential fat is found in the brain, nerves, bone marrow, heart tissue and cell walls. The amount of essential fat cannot be reduced without physiological functions being affected. Approximately 3 per cent of body weight in men and 12 per cent of body weight in women is essential fat. The higher percentage in women relates to reproduction and hormonal functions, and is found particularly in the pelvic and breast area. It is often called gender-specific fat.

Storage fat or adipose tissue is a major source of fuel. It is found under the skin (subcutaneous fat) and around the vital organs, where it has a protective function. The fat is stored in fat cells or adipocytes. Normally, fat cells contain about 45mg of fat but they are able to gain up to twice this amount. Women have considerably more storage fat than men. Again, the reasons for this are linked to reproduction, the difference in absolute terms being similar to the energy cost of pregnancy.

The whole body contains enough stored fat energy to keep the body alive for many weeks. When overweight and obese people lose weight, the amount of fat in the adipocytes drops but the actual number of adipocytes does not change. Reducing body fat towards

the point that there is essential body fat alone will impair physiological function and the capacity of the body to exercise, as well as causing certain health risks. It is generally accepted that the minimal body-fat level for men is not less than 5 per cent. There is no definitive minimal body-fat percentage for women, although ranges from 12 to 16 per cent have been quoted. An excessively low body fat or body weight in females should be avoided as it not only affects running performance but can have serious health implications (*see* Chapter 6). One thing is certain, essential fat percentage is definitely not optimal fat percentage.

Body Weight

For marathon runners body weight is the most important consideration in the power to weight ratio. A small body size means that the energy cost of running is lower. There may also be a thermoregulatory advantage as a smaller body is able to get rid of heat more easily and of course has less dead weight to carry around.

For many, the need to get fit and lose weight will be the incentive to start training to run a marathon. The simplest method of keeping a check on weight is to carry out regular weekly weighings. Conditions must always be the same – ideally, no shoes, minimal or no clothing, at the same time of day and using the same set of scales. The preferred and most convenient time is usually first thing in the morning before breakfast but after a successful visit to the lavatory. There can be daily fluctuations of up to 2 or more kg, particularly for women, so it is important not to become obsessed with the precise readings but to use them as an indication of the general trend in body weight. This is the main reason to discourage weighing more than once a week.

Standard height and weight charts can be misleading as they are usually based on the average weight of a sample population group and do not represent people who exercise regularly. With training there may be a loss of body fat and an increase in muscle mass. Muscle is a much denser tissue than fat so the same weight of fat takes up more space than the equivalent weight in muscle. Taking measurements with a tape measure or assessing looseness of previously tight clothing are rough but reasonable indicators of changes in body composition. Weight may stay the same but inches may be lost, indicating that body fat has gone down but muscle mass has increased. For some runners, an increase in weight may simply reflect dietary over-indulgence because training has been used as an excuse to over-eat!

MEASURING BMI AND BODY COMPOSITION

Body Mass Index

There is no ideal weight for all people of the same height, so using a *range* of values is more realistic. The body mass index (BMI), based on the relationship between height and weight, provides such a range. BMI is currently the internationally accepted standard for assessing how healthy or otherwise an individual's body weight is. However, it is not accurate for people who have a large muscle mass, as it can place them firmly but erroneously in an overweight category. Similarly, it is not accurate for those with a very low body fat, who may be placed incorrectly in a healthy category.

Body Composition

Measurement of body composition can be helpful in a variety of ways, particularly for monitoring desired changes, identifying health risks of runners with very low body fat levels and estimating ideal and minimal body weights for runners.

CALCULATING AND INTERPRETING BODY MASS INDEX (BMI)

BODY MASS INDEX (BMI) =

$$\frac{\text{Weight in kg}}{\text{Height} \times \text{Height in metres}}$$

For example: A male weighing 73kg and 1.85m tall would have a BMI of 21.3 (normal)

$$\text{BMI} = \frac{73\text{kg}}{1.85 \times 1.85} = 21.3$$

Classification	BMI
Underweight	<18.5
Normal	18.5–24.9
Overweight	25–29.9
Obese class I	30–34.9
Obese class II	35–39.9
Obese class III	>40

There are a variety of methods available for measuring body composition, including reference body composition methods, which are beyond the scope of this book. Field techniques (in other words, the more practical methods that can be used in gyms and running clubs) include measurements of skinfold thickness and bioelectrical impedance analysis (BIA).

Skinfold Thicknesses

This method involves the measurement of a fold of subcutaneous fat at one or more sites, which is then interpreted using equations to estimate fat mass. Generally, four sites are measured, although as many as twelve can be used. The triceps, biceps, subscapular and supra-iliac are the usual sites. Measurements are made using callipers, which exert a standardized pressure on the site that is being measured.

Skinfolds are probably the most widely used technique for estimating fat mass. This method has the advantage that it is non-invasive (although, depending on which sites are used, some degree of undressing may be necessary), costs little (once the callipers have been acquired) and can be used to highlight fat distribution (different parts of the body). There are disadvantages, too. Measurements are affected by the skill of the technician, the type of callipers used, the ease or otherwise of measuring the individual, and the accuracy of the prediction equations that are used to calculate the fat mass.

Bioelectrical Impedance Analysis (BIA)

In this method, a small current of electricity is passed between electrodes placed on the hands and feet. The voltage drop is measured to give an estimate of the body resistance or impedance. The current passes through the water and electrolyte component of lean tissue and, as the electrical resistance is proportional to the body water volume, this is then used to estimate lean body mass. Fat mass is then calculated by subtracting lean body mass from body weight.

This method is rapid, non-invasive and non-intrusive, relatively inexpensive and does not require any particular degree of technical skill. However, results are affected by the state of the runner at the time of measurement. Most accurate results will be obtained when the runner has not eaten or drunk anything for four hours, has not exercised during the last twelve hours, has not drunk alcohol in the last forty-eight hours and has not used diuretics in the last seven days. Urination must also have been achieved within the last thirty minutes. If these precautions are not taken each time a runner is measured, results could be misleading and the runner become unnecessarily disappointed or alternatively delighted by an inaccurate reading.

Not everyone has access to reliable scales, let alone other methods, so for many people the eye (or a tight pair of jeans) will give a rough but reasonable assessment of any changes. However, some individuals do have a distorted body self-image, believing that they are overweight or downright fat, when actually they are unhealthily thin.

If body fat measurements are taken, it is important that runners understand their limitations. There can be a large variation in body fat measurements depending on the method used. One study measuring body fat in ten competitive thirty-year-old male runners found that body fat ranged from 10.5 per cent with dual-energy X-ray absorptiometry (DEXA), 9 per cent with underwater weighing, 8.5 per cent with skinfold callipers and 6 per cent with bioelectrical impedance. Body fat measurements are most useful when assessed alongside other fitness tests so that a more complete picture of a runner's overall profile can be determined.

Ultimately, the most important indicator is the way a runner is performing. It is pointless battling to reach a lower body fat measurement if speed and stamina are dipping as a result.

CHAPTER 2
The Training Diet

A well-planned training diet will help to maximize training runs, aid recovery, reduce fatigue and keep the runner in good health. As weekly mileage goes up, and extra demands are placed on the carbohydrate stores, runners will find they have to adapt their diet, otherwise training will start to suffer. Training times may have to change and this can mean that different eating patterns and meal times have to be adopted. The weeks and months spent training for the marathon itself also provide an ideal opportunity to experiment with food and fluid intakes. As a result, when it comes to the actual marathon, a tried and tested diet and fluid strategy should be reassuringly in place.

ENERGY

Many runners will want to know what their approximate energy requirement is and how it changes as training progresses. Energy

---

CALCULATING THE BASAL METABOLIC RATE

BMR (MJ/day)

Age	BMR (males)	BMR (females)
10–17 years	0.074W + 2.754	0.056W + 2.898
18–29 years	0.063W + 2.896	0.062W + 2.036
30–39 years	0.048W + 3.653	0.034W + 3.538
60–74 years	0.0499W + 2.930	0.0386W + 2.875
75+ years	0.0350W + 3.434	0.041W + 2.610

BMR (kcal/day)

Age	BMR (males)	BMR (females)
10–17 years	17.7W + 657	13.4W + 692
18–29 years	15.1W + 692	14.8W + 487
30–59 years	11.5W + 873	8.3W + 846
60–74 years	11.9W + 700	9.2W + 687
75+ years	8.4W + 821	9.8W + 624

W = body weight (kg)

Reference: Schofield W.N., Scholfield C., James W.P.T., 'Basal metabolic rate – review and prediction', *Hum Nutr: Clin Nutr* (1985) 39 (suppl.), pp. 1–96.

expenditure (EE) is the sum of the basal metabolic rate (BMR) plus the cost of all the day's activities. The thermic effect of food and adaptive thermogenesis account for such a small proportion of the total energy expenditure that they can be discounted. Therefore, to work out an individual's energy requirement, the BMR must first be calculated, then the energy cost of everyday activities (which will be based mainly on type of work or otherwise) and, finally, the energy cost of running. This will give a reasonable indication of daily energy requirements.

The energy requirements of the working day are based on the physical activity level (PAL). If work is very sedentary (as in office work), this is given a PAL of 1.4 for men and women. If work is moderately active (as it is for medical workers, retail workers, students and transport workers), the PAL is 1.6 for men and 1.5 for women. Men involved in heavy work (for example, labourers, agricultural workers and those carrying out heavy construction work) should use a PAL of 1.7 and women involved in similar work, 1.5. To work out the daily requirements excluding the cost of running, the BMR is multiplied by the PAL. Finally the energy cost of running must be calculated. This depends on the distance covered and the body weight – body weight in kilograms, distance in kilometres and a factor of 1.036 are multiplied together. Many people take up running primarily to lose weight. As energy expenditure is partly dependent on body weight periodical recalculations will be needed as the weight falls.

It is not necessary for a runner to work out his or her energy requirements on a daily basis, neither is it suggested. One way to do it is to work out the energy cost of running on a weekly mileage and then to divide by seven to give a daily average. However, most people will actually match their requirement automatically with intake – led by a powerful hunger drive. Rather than working at the overall energy intake, it is more likely that runners will need to put thought into getting the *balance* of the main nutrients – carbohydrate, fat and protein – right.

CARBOHYDRATE

Although carbohydrate is the most important fuel for endurance running, the body's capacity to store it (as glycogen) is limited. Restoring

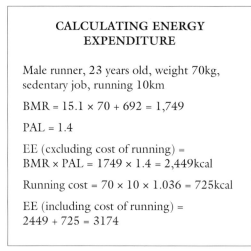

CALCULATING ENERGY EXPENDITURE

Male runner, 23 years old, weight 70kg, sedentary job, running 10km

BMR = 15.1 × 70 + 692 = 1,749

PAL = 1.4

EE (excluding cost of running) = BMR × PAL = 1749 × 1.4 = 2,449kcal

Running cost = 70 × 10 × 1.036 = 725kcal

EE (including cost of running) = 2449 + 725 = 3174

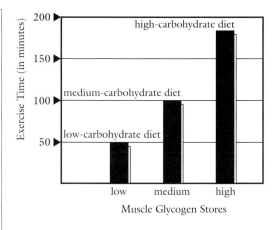

Effect of diet on glycogen stores and exercise time.

depleted glycogen levels in the muscles between training runs can only be achieved by eating a high-carbohydrate diet on a regular basis.

An increase in mileage can cause temporary feelings of tiredness but these soon disappear as the runner adapts to a new workload. Symptoms of fatigue caused by a low carbohydrate intake include muscle heaviness, poor energy levels in training, a feeling of great effort but without the expected outcome, and progressive tiredness over the week. Low carbohydrate intake may not be the only cause of tiredness. Fatigue may also be related to a long-term poor intake of iron in the diet. Other causes could be a dramatic increase in weekly mileage, which can be remedied by cutting back the number of miles run, and insufficient recovery time between runs; running *quality* is just as important as the number of miles covered each week. Other significant factors include lack of sleep or a generally exhausting lifestyle, but poor nutrition is usually to blame.

Although many runners recognize the importance of a high-carbohydrate diet, their own diet often contains no more than that of the general public, which will certainly not be enough. Figures from *The National Diet and Nutrition Survey: Adults aged 19 to 64 years*, published in the UK in 2003, revealed that mean daily intake of total carbohydrate was 275g for men and 203g for women, an average of 48 per cent of total energy. This is considerably less than the requirements for someone training to run a marathon.

Carbohydrate Intake

Levels

Carbohydrate recommendations for the general public are often given as a percentage of total energy. Even for athletes, percentages of 55 to 70 per cent are still quoted. Relating carbohydrate to body weight is a much more accurate and useful way of calculating carbohydrate

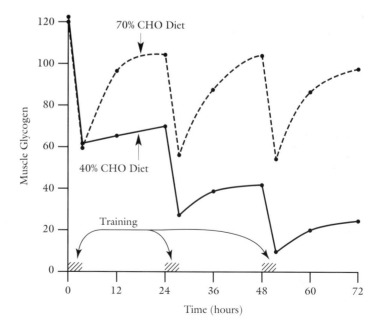

Replacement of muscle glycogen after prolonged daily training sessions.

SOURCE: D. L. Costill and J. M. Miller; *International Journal of Sports Medicine* 1:2–14 (1980)

ESTIMATED DAILY CARBOHYDRATE REQUIREMENTS	
Time spent running	Requirement g per kg body weight per day
3 to 5 hours a week	4 to 5g carbohydrate
5 to 7 hours a week	5 to 6g carbohydrate
1 to 2 hours a day	6 to 7g carbohydrate
2 to 4 hours a day	7 to 8g carbohydrate
4+ hours a day	8 to 10g carbohydrate

requirements as it takes into account not only the different intakes of men and women but also the different levels of training intensity. In other words, it relates more to the muscles' absolute needs for fuel. Armed with information about the carbohydrate content of different foods, runners should be able to add more carbohydrate into the diet to match the requirements of an increasing weekly mileage.

Timing

The time when carbohydrate is eaten is also important. Rates of muscle glycogen storage are fastest in the first two hours after a run, after which the rate slows to the normal typical rate. If a runner fails to have carbohydrate during this period, glycogen replacement will be slower. This could have an impact on any running undertaken the next day. Effective glycogen replacement will occur regardless of whether the carbohydrate intake is in the form of drinks, snacks or a meal. What matters is that carbohydrate is provided in sufficient amounts. Within the first two hours, 1 to 1.2g carbohydrate per kilogram body weight is needed and consumption must begin as early as possible. The carbohydrate requirement for immediate refuelling is included in the total twenty-four-hour requirement. It is not *additional*.

In the early stages of training, when mileage is low and there is at least twenty-four hours between runs, the timing is less crucial. Refuelling and meals can be organized to take place when the runner feels comfortable eating, and to fit into the normal daily routine.

It is important to avoid foods with a high fat content as these can suppress appetite and, consequently, limit carbohydrate intake. This is particularly important if a runner is going to eat a meal rather than a snack immediately after running. Appetite can be suppressed after running, especially if the weather is warm. Taste sensation after exercise often veers towards a preference for sweet-tasting foods.

The Glycaemic Index

Identifying GI

The glycaemic index of carbohydrate foods offers great opportunities for the runner in terms of providing carbohydrate at different rates, depending on whether it is pre-, during or post-exercise. However, one of the drawbacks of the GI is that numerous factors can influence the GI of a food, let alone a meal. These include portion size (hence the introduction of the glycaemic load), whether the item is cooked or raw, the particular cooking method used, presence of any fat, and the overall size of the meal. Originally, it was thought that complex or starchy carbohydrate foods, such as bread, rice, pasta and potatoes were digested more slowly, causing a gradual increase in blood-sugar levels. In fact, starchy foods are actually digested very rapidly and absorbed quickly. On the other hand, moderate amounts of many sugary foods do not generally produce the dramatic rise in blood sugar that had previously been assumed. Foods containing sucrose actually show quite low-to-moderate blood-glucose responses, lower than foods such as rice.

For runners needing to know more information about the glycaemic index of particular foods, there are many diet and nutrition books. The *International table of glycemic index and glycemic load values: 2002* contains 1,300 data entries derived from published and unpublished verified sources, representing more than 750 different types of foods (Foster-Powell, K., Holt, S., Brand-Miller, J.C., *Am J.Clin.Nutr.* 2002; 76:5–56). The GI is becoming a popular concept and numerous books on the subject, particularly relating to weight loss, can be found on bookshelves. Some supermarkets have had products tested by Oxford Brookes University and now incorporate labels indicating 'low-GI' or 'medium-GI'.

Glycaemic Index and Performance

Low- to moderate-GI foods should be used before running as they will provide a more sustained source of carbohydrate. Consuming carbohydrate during long training runs and the marathon itself can help to top up the progressively depleting stores of muscle glycogen and therefore prolong the onset of fatigue and the resulting dip in exercise capacity and performance. Whatever is consumed during exercise must be easily digested and absorbed and therefore available to provide a rapid source of energy. No runner will want to have the sensation of something in the stomach, either.

Moderate- and high-GI items will be the best choice both during and immediately after running, when rapid refuelling is needed. The GI may lead the runner to favour one food or drink over another, but it is just one factor to be considered. The nutritional balance, taste and practicality of the food must also be taken into consideration. Runners must feel comfortable with the drinks and foods that they have before, during and after running. Interestingly, a breakfast of bacon and egg has an extremely low GI because it has almost no carbohydrates, but it is surely not the ideal choice for a pre-run meal!

Sugar and Exercise

Runners are often advised to avoid sugar before running. This is based on research carried out over two decades ago, which showed that consuming 75g of glucose (300kcal) thirty minutes before exercise reduced cycling time to exhaustion. The researchers suggested that glucose caused the pancreas to secrete a lot of insulin, which lowered the blood-sugar level and pushed the glucose into the muscles. The

---

GLYCAEMIC INDEX OF SOME COMMON FOODS

Low-GI foods (GI less than 55):
noodles, pasta, basmati rice, lentils, apples and apple juice, pears, oranges and orange juice, grapes, bananas, dried apricots, milk, low-fat yoghurt, fruit loaf, baked beans, porridge, 'fruit and fibre'-type cereals, pitta bread, granary and multigrain bread.

Intermediate-GI foods (GI 55–70):
new and boiled potatoes, macaroni, couscous, pineapple, sultanas and raisins, fibre-enriched white bread, oatmeal biscuits, honey.

High-GI foods (GI more than 70):
instant and mashed potato, jacket potatoes and chips, brown and white rice, parsnips, swede, broad beans and watermelon, cornflakes, Weetabix, Shredded Wheat, Rice Krispies, brown, wholemeal and white bread, bagels, crumpets and rice cakes, jelly babies and jelly beans.

GI index is certainly not predictable!

glucose level was further lowered when the muscles began to use blood glucose at the start of exercise. The overall lowering of blood sugar was thought to be responsible for the fatigue and subsequent drop in endurance performance that was observed.

Recent studies have shown that, despite the rise in insulin levels at the beginning of exercise and a fall in glucose concentration during exercise, all as a result of pre-exercise intake of glucose, blood-glucose concentration returned to normal as exercise continued. There was also no detrimental effect on performance from very low blood-glucose levels. It is suggested that this may be because the drop in blood-glucose concentration was either too brief or too small. However, hypoglycaemia may occur with prolonged exercise as the runner becomes fatigued and eventually even exhausted. This hypoglycaemia is associated with depletion of liver and muscle glycogen stores so that energy cannot be produced quickly enough.

Even so, a very small number of runners are sensitive to low blood-glucose concentrations and aware of feeling fatigued. Such runners would do well to avoid glucose intake in the hour before they start running. Carbohydrate consumed during exercise provides an extra source of fuel for the exercising muscles. It does not seem to change the rate of utilization of muscle glycogen but it does provide more fuel as blood glucose.

Hypoglycaemia

Normally, the movement of blood glucose into the muscles after ingestion of a meal or snack is very finely controlled by the production of the right amount of insulin to bring the blood-glucose level back to normal. In a very small percentage of the general population, the blood-sugar level returns to normal very quickly after eating, so fast that more insulin is produced than is needed. As a result,

more sugar is removed from the bloodstream, causing the level to drop below normal, leading to hypoglycaemia or low blood glucose. Many of the symptoms of hypoglycaemia are similar to those often related to stress, such as sweating, palpitations, anxiety and weakness. Others may include bad temper and poor concentration. A true diagnosis can only be made by a blood test carried out when the symptoms are actually present – when the blood-glucose level would be expected to be low.

Athletes who are medically diagnosed with hypoglycaemia should eat regular meals and never miss breakfast, particularly if they are running early in the morning. They should try to eat at least every three hours and include low-GI carbohydrate foods at all meals and snack occasions. High-GI carbohydrate-rich foods should not be eaten alone as a snack. They should be mixed with low-GI carbohydrate foods to give an overall moderate GI.

Building Up Carbohydrate Intake

There are a wide variety of suitable carbohydrate foods that can be included in a marathon runner's diet but there may be a tendency to build the diet around a limited number of foods – for example, the same breakfast cereal, or the same sandwiches using the same bread. Healthy messages directed at the general public, such as the advice to include more dietary fibre, are not always appropriate for those who have a high physical activity level. Wholegrain cereals, wholemeal bread, brown rice and so on, are all filling foods and could limit overall consumption so that carbohydrate requirements are not met.

To keep the diet interesting, runners should open their eyes to the huge variety of carbohydrate-containing foods that are available and, instead of buying the same bread or breakfast cereal every time, experiment and try something new.

TYPICAL HIGH CARBOHYDRATE INTAKE
TO MATCH A HIGH WEEKLY MILEAGE

Breakfast:
- glass of fruit juice (orange, grapefruit, apple and so on);
- bowl of breakfast cereal of choice with added dried fruit or sliced banana and semi-skimmed milk;
- toast (white bread if preferred) with a spread (butter, polyunsaturated or monounsaturated margarine or low-fat spread) and jam, honey or marmalade;
- tea, coffee, hot chocolate or water to drink.

Mid-morning:
- fruit bun, scone or malt loaf;
- hot or cold drink.

Lunch:
- sandwiches, rolls, baps or bagels with a spread (as Breakfast) and a suitable filling of chicken, ham, lean beef, tuna, salmon, egg or cheese.
- Include salad vegetables in the sandwich or in a separate box;
- piece of fruit or some dried fruit;
- pot of low-fat yoghurt or rice pudding;
- hot or cold drink.

Mid-afternoon:
- cereal or breakfast bar or dried fruit and nuts;
- hot or cold drink.

Evening meal:
- pasta, rice, potatoes (jacket, boiled or mashed);
- chicken, fish, lean meat, pulses (lentils, beans and so on) or Quorn, soya or tofu;
- two vegetables;
- fruit, yoghurt or a simple pudding, such as apple crumble or sponge with custard or ice-cream;
- water or fruit juice.

Late-evening refueller
(if still hungry before bed):
- toast or a bowl of cereal with milk;
- hot chocolate or hot milk.

Snacking is often seen as something to be avoided. Again, this may be appropriate advice for sedentary individuals but, for runners with high energy and carbohydrate requirements, eating little and often rather than having large infrequent meals is often the only way to meet requirements. It is not a crime to eat between meals and adopt a grazing eating pattern. Rather than referring to 'snacking', it can be called 'fuelling' or 'eating a mini-meal' instead.

Meeting Carbohydrate Requirements

For some runners, particularly novice runners at the very beginning of their marathon training programme, the advice given so far will be enough to ensure that glycogen stores are maintained. Others who train regularly, and novices in time, will want to know how to ensure that they are meeting their total requirement for the mileage they are doing, including the amount for refuelling immediately after each run. Equipped with information about portions of food and drink that provide 50g of carbohydrate, and the carbohydrate content of refuelling items (by reading food labels), such as cereal and breakfast bars and some confectionery, cakes and biscuits, and of course sports drinks, the runner can build up the total daily carbohydrate intake

---

GOOD SOURCES OF CARBOHYDRATE

Breakfast cereals: any variety (it doesn't have to be wholegrain), including hot cereals such as porridge. Many varieties can be eaten dry as a quick snack.
Bread: all types, including bagels, English muffins, crumpets, pikelets, naans, chappatis, potato cakes, raisin bread, malt loaf, fruit loaf, rye bread, tea breads, pancakes, tortillas and wraps, soft pretzels.
Crispbreads, water biscuits, oatcakes, crackers, rice cakes and matzos.
Pasta and noodles.
Rice.
Polenta, couscous, bulgur wheat, millet and quinoa.
Potatoes, sweet potatoes, yam, cassava, plantains.
Pizza bases.
Beans: baked, butter, red kidney, chickpeas, barlotti, cannelloni and mixed.
Peas, lentils, pearl barley.
Sweetcorn and popcorn (preferably salted not buttered).
Root vegetables: carrots, parsnips, swedes, turnips, sweet potatoes, beetroot.

Fruit: fresh, dried, canned, cooked.
Jam, marmalade, honey, fruit spreads, golden syrup, maple syrup, molasses, black treacle.
Twiglets, sesame sticks, Japanese rice crackers, breadsticks, pretzels.
Biscuits: Jaffa Cakes, fig rolls, garibaldi, rich tea, plain digestives.
Cakes: currant buns, iced fruit buns, Chelsea buns, plain or fruit scones, fruit cake, gingerbread, parkin, jam-filled Swiss roll, flapjacks, cake bars and other similar 'simple or plain' cakes.
Breakfast, cereal and muesli bars.
Puddings: fruit crumbles, bread pudding, milk puddings (for example, rice pudding), jelly and custard, banana and custard, meringue.
Yoghurt: fruit and natural.
Milk, milk shakes and smoothies.
Sweetened soft drinks: squash, cordial, canned drinks.
Fruit juice and vegetable juice.
Confectionery: chocolate bars and sweets.
Sugar: added to drinks and breakfast cereals.
Sports products: drinks, bars and gels.

---

as well as satisfying the specific requirements for refuelling after training runs, races and the marathon itself.

Eating Before Running

Food consumed before running is only useful once it is digested and absorbed. A general guide is to have a meal three or four hours before running and a small, light meal or snack about one to two hours before. The actual timing can only be determined by trial and error on the part of the runner. Finding what feels comfortable will be an enormous benefit when it comes to race days. Gut contents do get moved around in running so it is

important to get it right. Foods should be chosen primarily for their carbohydrate content, not only because of the fuel value but also because carbohydrate is digested and absorbed more quickly than other nutrients. Pre-run foods should therefore also be low in fat and fibre.

Carbohydrate Intake During Running

This topic is covered in detail in Chapter 3. It is worth mentioning here that, although taking on board carbohydrate while running helps to boost the limited stores of carbohydrate in the body, recent research suggests that it may have another benefit. In this particular

SUITABLE PRE-RUN FOODS

3–4 hours before running:
- toast or crumpets with jam or honey and a milk shake;
- baked beans on toast;
- bowl of cereal and low-fat milk with a banana;
- bowl of fruit salad with low-fat yoghurt;
- sandwiches with a low-fat spread and filling such as chicken, lean ham, tuna or low-fat soft cheese;
- pasta or rice with a low-fat sauce such as tomato, vegetables, very lean meat.

1–2 hours before running:
- milk shake or smoothie;
- cereal bar, breakfast bar or sports bar;
- bowl of cereal and low-fat milk;
- low-fat yoghurt or rice;
- fruit.

Less than 1 hour before running:
- sports drink;
- gel;
- sports bar;
- jelly sweets.

FOOD DURING THE RACE

Suitable foods while running include the following:

- boiled sweets, fruit pastilles, jelly or jelly sweets;
- bananas;
- dried fruit, for example, raisins, dates, apricots;
- sports bars;
- not everybody's choice, but marzipan is suitable!

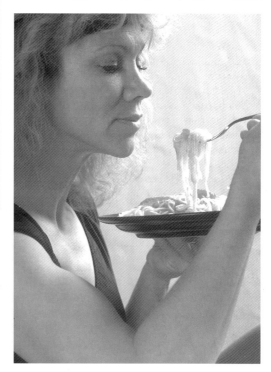

Woman eating pasta. (GETTY IMAGES)

study, during a marathon, runners given carbo-hydrate supplements were able to maintain their running at a higher percentage of their maximum heart rate; in other words, they were able to run at a higher intensity, despite the fact that their perception of exertion was not significantly different from that of the control group. The major contribution to carbohydrate intake will almost certainly come from the use of a sports drink.

Carbohydrate Intake After Running

Ideally, refuelling should start within fifteen minutes of finishing, even taking priority over a shower. Between 1 and 1.2g of carbohydrate per kg body weight should be consumed as either fluids or a combination of fluids and foods. This should then be followed, if possible,

---

FOOD AFTER THE RACE

Suitable refuelling items for immediately after running include the following:

- sports drinks, gels and bars;
- cereal and breakfast bars*
  (but not flapjacks);
- toast and honey;
- pancakes and syrup;
- thick vegetable soup and bread or rolls;
- rice pudding;
- Twiglets* (but not crisps);
- Jaffa Cakes* (but not chocolate).

* Because they contain less fat.

---

by some more food or a meal within the next two hours. High-GI foods will help to refuel fastest but it is just as important to find carbohydrate-rich foods and fluids that are appropriate in other ways; most importantly, they must be palatable and give the runner enjoyment at the end of a hard training run or race.

Gels and Sports Bars

There are a variety of gels and sports or energy bars on the market, and some runners might find it useful to carry some in a bum bag on longer runs and races. Gels are easier to carry than the heavier and bigger bars and most runners find they are also easy to swallow while running. They contain a high concentration of carbohydrate so it is important to drink plenty of water at the same time. Instructions on the pack should indicate how much fluid needs to be drunk per gel. Runners should work out at home exactly how much this fluid is *in mouthfuls*, so that they know exactly how many mouthfuls they need per sachet or pouch while running. Not drinking enough could cause dehydration

because fluid is drawn into the stomach to dilute the carbohydrate.

Sports bars also provide a compact supply of carbohydrate and protein and are usually (and should be) low in fat and fibre. They are designed for easy eating, speedy digestion and are suitable for eating both during and immediately after running. Like many specialist foods, they can be expensive; certainly, they tend to cost more than cereal or breakfast bars. As they deliver more carbohydrate and protein than conventional bars, it would seem sensible to limit their use to longer training runs and races. As with the gels, sports bars will need to be eaten with some water. This will aid swallowing (particularly if the mouth has become dry) and digestion. Most runners will find that eating small amounts at a time is more enjoyable and certainly more comfortable than eating a whole bar in one go. The bars can be quite heavy to carry while running, which is another factor to consider.

FAT

Fat is needed in the diet. It has many important functions and runners should never attempt to follow a 'no-fat' diet. However, in order to achieve the required intake of carbohydrate and protein, while maintaining body weight, it will be necessary to ensure a low intake of fat. Most runners will be able to do this by learning which foods contain a relatively large amount of fat and by following simple practical guidelines.

Some foods that are high in fat can also be a very good source of essential nutrients – cheese is a very good example. It is therefore important not to exclude such items from the diet but rather to use smaller portions or look for low-fat varieties. This is particularly important for those who are running to lose weight. Overall intakes must not be reduced

A HIGH-FAT VERSUS A LOW-FAT MENU

	Full-fat menu	Fat (g)	Reduced-fat menu	Fat (g)
Breakfast	Bowl of cornflakes		Bowl of cornflakes	
	Full-cream milk	4	Semi-skimmed milk	2
	Slice white toast		Slice white toast, low-fat spread,	
	Butter and marmalade	8	marmalade	2
Mid-morning	Mars bar	12	Banana	
	Cup of coffee	1	Glass of juice	
Lunch	Cheese and pickle sandwich	33	Lean ham and tomato sandwich	6
	Packet of crisps	10	Piece of fruit	
	2 chocolate biscuits	11	Tea cake and low-fat spread	8
Mid-afternoon Snack	Cereal crunchy bar	7	2 digestive biscuits	6
Evening meal	2 fried sausages	20	2 reduced-fat grilled sausages	11
	Chips	11	Jacket potato	
	Peas		Salad	
	Apple crumble and full-fat custard	17	Apple crumble and custard with semi-skimmed milk	12
	Total	**134**		**47**

to the point where training is compromised. A nutritionally well-balanced energy-controlled diet plus training is the safest and most effective way to lose weight.

A Role for High-Fat Diets?

There is no good evidence that a high-fat/low-carbohydrate diet can improve performance (with perhaps the exception of the ultra-endurance runner). Fat can be utilized in low-intensity exercise but fat oxidation cannot supply energy fast enough when exercise intensity is greater than about 60 per cent VO_2max

(in other words, moderate-intensity exercise). Eating too much fat also tends to decrease carbohydrate intake so that muscle glycogen stores are not maintained satisfactorily. Alternatively, if sufficient carbohydrate is consumed along with a high-fat diet, overall energy intake will certainly be in excess of energy requirements, leading to an increase in body fat.

From a health point of view, high-fat diets are associated with heart disease, stroke, some forms of cancer and, of course, overweight and obesity. High-fat diets suppress some aspects of immune function compared to carbohydrate-rich diets. However, a moderate

OMEGA-3 CONTENT OF FISH

	g per 100g portion
Salmon, Atlantic, farmed, cooked, dry heat	1.8
Sardines, canned in tomato sauce, drained	1.4
Herring, Atlantic, pickled	1.2
Mackerel, Atlantic, cooked, dry heat	1.0
Trout, rainbow, farmed, cooked, dry heat	1.0
Swordfish, cooked, dry heat	0.7
Tuna, white, canned in water, drained	0.7
Cod, Atlantic, cooked, dry heat	0.1

amount of omega-3 polyunsaturated fatty acids can be beneficial to the immune system. This can be achieved simply by including oily fish in the weekly diet. Unfortunately, the majority of the population does not eat much oily fish. Current average adult intakes are 53g per week yet recommendations for general health point to at least 280g a week (equivalent to two portions). Girls under sixteen years of age, pregnant women or those who may become pregnant, and breastfeeding women should have no more than this amount; other populations can have up to four portions.

Fat loading is claimed to help a runner burn fat and spare glycogen, which, in turn, can enhance endurance capacity. Human studies have shown that ingestion of a high-fat diet for three to five days leads to a deterioration in endurance performance compared to a high-carbohydrate diet. From one to four weeks, a high-fat diet in combination with training does not reduce endurance performance compared with a high-carbohydrate diet but neither does it improve it. After seven weeks on the regime, endurance performance was markedly better on the high-carbohydrate diet compared to the high-fat diet. In addition, high-fat diets take longer to digest, hence the need to avoid high-fat foods in a pre-exercise meal.

Similarly, there seems to be no benefit gained when an athlete switches to a high-carbohydrate diet after a long-term adaptation to a high-fat diet, compared to having a high-carbohydrate intake all along. Aerobic training, of course, does increase a runner's ability to utilize intramuscular triglycerides (fat stored directly within the muscle fibres) as a source of fuel. This helps to extend the more limited carbohydrate reserves and enables the runner to continue for longer.

PROTEIN

Protein Requirements

Protein requirements for distance runners are related to the duration and intensity of exercise, as well as to gender, age, training status and energy and carbohydrate intake. As mileage increases and glycogen stores become depleted, protein is used to provide a small proportion of the energy costs of training. At the end of a marathon, females may be meeting 2 per cent of their energy needs by metabolizing protein and males up to 6 per cent. Initially, novice runners or first-time marathon runners will need proportionately more protein than well-trained endurance runners. This is because there is an extra protein requirement, to cover the cost of the increase in muscle mass, red blood

REDUCING FAT IN THE DIET

- Use semi-skimmed or skimmed milk.
- Use low-fat yoghurts, fromage frais and quark.
- Keep cream to occasional use only. Use low-fat soft cheese to make a 'creamy' sauce.
- Use lower-fat cheeses or less of a strongly flavoured full-fat one.
- Grate cheese to make it go further.
- Buy fish canned in brine, water or tomatoes rather than oil.
- Avoid all poultry skin as most fat is under the skin.
- Buy lean meat and trim off visible fat.
- Drain off fat from meat juices when making gravy, or use a gravy pourer.
- Use low-fat spreads rather than butter or margarine.
- Skip the fat spread altogether, particularly if using tasty continental breads or having baked beans on toast.
- Microwave, steam, poach, boil, grill or stir-fry rather than frying.
- Use non-stick pans or a spray oil.
- 'Roast' potatoes by parboiling, brushing lightly with oil and crisping in a pre-heated oven.
- Keep chips occasional. Best choice is low-fat, thick, straight oven chips.
- Avoid pastry items such as meat pies, sausage rolls and pasties. Filo pastry and crumbles are the best way to satisfy an urge for pastry.
- Check food labels carefully. Make sure that low-fat products are also lower in energy than the traditional version.

FOOD PORTIONS PROVIDING APPROX 20G PROTEIN

Food	Quantity of food	Portion of food
Beef, lamb, pork	75g	2 medium slices
Chicken	75g	1 small breast
Fish (cod, haddock etc.)	100g	1 medium fillet
Salmon	100g	1 average steak
Mackerel	100g	1 small smoked fillet
Fish fingers	135g	5 fingers
Tuna in brine	100g	1 small can
Prawns, boiled (no shell)	100g	approx 30 small prawns
Semi/skimmed milk	600ml	1 pint
Skimmed milk powder	40g	4 tablespoons
Cheddar cheese, reduced fat	60g	2 matchbox-sized pieces
Low-fat fruit yoghurt	400g	2 × 200g pots (Müllerlight)
Eggs		3 size 2 eggs
Baked beans	400g	1 large can
Lentils, cooked or canned	265g	6½ tablespoons
Chickpeas, cooked or canned	270g	7½ tablespoons
Red kidney beans, cooked or canned	290g	8 tablespoons
Soya mince	46g	3 tablespoons
Brazil or walnuts	140g	20 whole nuts
Quorn mince	165g	6½ tablespoons
Tofu, steamed	250g	

cells, myoglobin and enzymes needed for metabolism. Current general recommendations for protein intake, set at 0.75g protein per kg body weight per day, are based on a sedentary lifestyle. Recommendations for endurance athletes are 1.2–1.4g per kg body weight per day.

The extra protein needs of runners can be met quite simply by including a wide variety of foods and eating food to meet energy requirements. Many sources of vegetable protein (peas, beans, lentils and nuts) contain large amounts of carbohydrate, dietary fibre, vitamins and minerals, as well as protein, and these foods should be included perhaps more often than in the normal course of events. Foods included in the diet primarily for their carbohydrate content also make a significant contribution to the overall protein intake, not so much because they are a rich protein source, but because they are eaten in such large amounts. For example, four slices of bread, eight tablespoons of cooked pasta or twelve tablespoons of cooked rice will each provide 10g protein. Protein supplements are definitely not needed in a marathon runner's daily diet.

Protein and Recovery

Recent studies have shown that when protein as well as carbohydrate is consumed immediately after exercise, not only are glycogen stores replenished more quickly, but there is also a marked uptake of amino acids by the muscles. Compared to carbohydrate, only a small amount of protein appears to be needed, probably as little as 15–20g. A chicken sandwich, tuna or cottage cheese with a jacket potato, baked beans on toast or a large milk shake or smoothie would all be simple practical ways of achieving the correct balance of protein and carbohydrate.

VITAMIN SUPPLEMENTS

Many runners regularly take vitamin supplements throughout training and competition, in the mistaken belief that extra vitamins improve performance. Many B vitamins are involved in the release of energy from carbohydrate and fat but there is no evidence that taking supplements on top of a perfectly adequate diet will release energy faster or enhance performance. Folate and vitamin B_{12} are important in red blood cell formation but taking extra will not stimulate the production of more red blood cells. If there is a vitamin deficiency because requirements are not being met, then health as well as performance will suffer. Taking a supplement to correct the deficiency and then ensuring that the diet provides enough to meet requirements will result in an improvement in both health and performance. Taking extra vitamins on top of a well-balanced diet will not enhance performance further.

Many runners experience tiredness, lethargy or heaviness in the legs and assume this to be caused by lack of vitamins. Inadequate energy, carbohydrate and/or fluid intakes and lack of rest days are the more likely culprits. In all these cases, reaching for a supplement will not provide the answer; implementing appropriate changes to the diet and including rest days will make a difference.

An increased requirement might be caused by decreased absorption by the digestive system, increased excretion in sweat, urine and faeces, increased turnover, as well as via a biochemical adaptation to training. In fact, there is little evidence to suggest that runners excrete more vitamins in urine and faeces or have a higher turnover of vitamins than inactive people. Even vitamin loss through sweat is negligible. The 'assumed' increased requirements are most likely to be the result of biochemical adaptations to training. In most

POSSIBLE CAUSES OF INADEQUATE VITAMIN INTAKES

Heavy reliance on convenience food and take-away meals.

Poor intake of fresh fruit and vegetables.

Regular meal skipping, due to lack of time to shop, cook or even eat.

Fussy eating.

Drug use interfering with vitamin metabolism, for example, contraceptive pill, aspirin and other anti-inflammatory drugs.

Vegan diet.

Excessive alcohol intake.

Regular smoking.

situations, this increased requirement will be met by the diet alone but not always.

The possible causes of inadequate intake tend to be lifestyle issues rather than runners having greater requirements compared to less active people. Although a supplement providing no more than 100 per cent of the Recommended Daily Amount (RDA) will never replace a healthy, well-balanced, varied diet or make up for a poor one, it can help to reduce nutritional gaps in the diet. A supplement providing 100 per cent (or less) of the RDA is the best choice for topping up the diet or even just to take as an insurance policy.

Runners should not combine different supplements without first seeking advice from their doctor, pharmacist or sports dietitian. Combining supplements can lead to megadosing, which can result in harmful side-effects. The supplement probably needs to be taken only every two or three days rather than every day. It is definitely not better to take any more than the amount recommended on the

pack by the manufacturer or retailer. The time of day when supplements are taken is not important but they should be taken regularly. Many runners find it best to get into a routine, for example, always having the supplement with breakfast and keeping it by the cereal box as a reminder.

Supplements containing vitamin B_2 (riboflavin) can cause a runner to produce bright-yellow urine. This can have implications when using urine colour as a sign of hydration status.

MINERALS

Minerals are essential nutrients that must be supplied in the diet. With the exception of calcium and iron, deficiencies are uncommon. Other minerals may be lost from the body during training but these will normally be replaced by a varied diet that is meeting energy requirements. Calcium and iron present specific problems because the best dietary sources are sometimes foods that are excluded from the diet for a variety of reasons, some valid, others based on misconceptions and misinformation.

Calcium

Almost 90 per cent of calcium is found in the bones. Bone is an active tissue, constantly changing as the result of the continual process of bone resorption and bone formation. Peak bone mass is the highest bone mass that is achieved in a person's lifetime and it is normally reached by the early thirties. After this time, bone mass begins to fall with age as resorption starts to exceed formation slightly. The rate of decline in bone mass with age is similar, regardless of the peak bone mass achieved, so having a high peak bone mass will help to prevent or at least delay the onset of osteoporosis or brittle-bone disease in later life. As weight-bearing exercise exerts an anabolic effect on the skeleton, bone density is usually higher in runners, particularly at the sites being exercised. For runners, this will be the calcaneum (heel bone), tibia (shin bone), femur (thigh bone) and spine.

Calcium in the Diet

Dairy products are the best source of calcium, but fear of fat in the diet has led many runners to cut dairy foods out of their diet. Oddly, semi-skimmed and skimmed milk actually contain slightly more calcium than full-fat milk. This is because the majority of the minerals and vitamins are found in the non-fat part of milk (with, of course, the exception of the fat-soluble vitamins). Calcium in vegetables and high-fibre foods may not be as easily absorbed as that in milk. Runners who restrict food intake to maintain a low body weight may be at particular risk if their diet is habitually low in calcium.

Practical Ways to Increase Calcium Intake

One of the easiest ways to ensure an adequate intake is to consume '3-a-Day': an average glass (200ml) of semi-skimmed or skimmed milk, a small pot (150g) of low-fat yoghurt and a matchbox-sized (40g) piece of cheese. Having milk or yoghurt with breakfast cereal every morning can boost the absorption of calcium from cereal, too. Other simple ways to boost intake include adding grated cheese to salads, soups and home-made pizzas, sprinkling sesame or sunflower seeds on salads and cooked vegetables, using yoghurt-based dressings on salads, and topping jacket potatoes with natural yoghurt and chives. Porridge can be made with milk rather than water. Custard made with milk can be enjoyed with fruit, alone, or as a frozen dessert. Mashing up canned salmon or sardines, including the calcium-rich bones, with lemon juice provides a variation on tuna for a sandwich

GOOD SOURCES OF CALCIUM IN THE DIET

Dairy produce

1 pint whole milk	673mg
1 pint semi-skimmed milk	702mg
1 pint skimmed milk	702mg
Matchbox-sized piece of Cheddar (40g)	288mg
Matchbox-sized piece low-fat Cheddar (40g)	336mg
4oz/100g cottage cheese	73mg
5oz/150g pot fruit yoghurt	225mg

Cereals

2 large slices white or brown bread	80mg
2 large slices wholemeal bread	39mg

Fish (plus bones)

100g can sardines in tomato sauce	460mg

Vegetables and pulses

3 'spears' of broccoli (150g)	50mg
Quarter of a bunch watercress	34mg
2 tablespoons (90g) cooked spinach	144mg
225g can baked beans in tomato sauce	120mg
Average serving tofu (bean curd)	306mg

Nuts

100g bag plain peanuts	60mg
1 tablespoon sesame seeds	80mg

Fruit

12 ready to eat dried apricots	73mg
1 large orange	50mg

Ice-cream

1 scoop dairy ice-cream	78mg

filling. Baked beans can be used as a vegetable, not just for beans on toast. Refuelling after a run with dried apricots will also boost calcium intake as will milk shakes and smoothies made with milk, yoghurt and fruit. A mug of hot chocolate at bedtime, made with milk, can give a final boost to the day's intake.

IRON

Iron is found in haemoglobin in the red blood cells, in myoglobin in the muscle cell and in some of the oxidative enzymes in the mitochondria (the energy-producing factories in the cells). A shortage of iron will therefore have a serious effect on energy metabolism. A deficiency of iron is accompanied by common symptoms such as chronic fatigue, susceptibility to stress, increased susceptibility to infections and decreased cognitive performance. Sub-optimal iron status is one of the most common nutritional problems found in the general community and the athletic population group seems to be no exception in this respect.

Runners have several risk factors for anaemia and iron depletion, some of which occur in the general population and some of which are unique to them.

RISK FACTORS FOR ANAEMIA AND IRON DEPLETION

Poor iron intakes.
Foot strike haemolysis (*see* Chapter 7).
Gastrointestinal bleeding.
Small iron losses in sweat.
Menstrual losses in females.

Iron Status and Performance

Iron depletion (identified by reduced serum ferritin levels) is not associated with a fall in exercise performance. In iron deficiency, red blood cell formation is impaired and haemoglobin levels begin to fall towards the lower end of the acceptable range. Again, running does not appear to be affected at this stage, but, if the situation continues, iron deficiency anaemia eventually develops. This will have a negative effect on performance. Iron supplements will correct the iron deficiency anaemia and restore performance levels.

Taking iron supplements when there is no iron deficiency anaemia present, even if iron depletion or non-anaemic iron deficiency are present, will not have any effect on performance. Runners should be cautious if they donate blood. Fluid is made up within hours but restoration of red blood cells to normal levels takes three or more weeks.

Iron in the Diet

There are two types of iron in the diet. Haem iron is found in meat and meat products and non-haem iron is found in cereals, vegetables, peas, beans and lentils, and fruits. Haem iron is well absorbed by the body, with up to 20 to 40 per cent being taken up, whereas only 5 to 20 per cent of iron from vegetable sources, egg and milk is absorbed. Many runners avoid meat because of the perceived fat content. In fact, due to a combination of breeding, feed changes and modern butchery techniques, the fat content of lean red meat has fallen by about a third over the last twenty years. A runner may choose not to eat meat for a variety of reasons but fat content is not a valid one.

GOOD SOURCES OF IRON IN THE DIET

Food (portion)	Iron per portion (mg)	Food (portion)	Iron per portion (mg)
		Rice, cooked av portion (4½ tbsp)	0.4mg
Animal sources			
2 slices liver (100g)	9mg	*Vegetables and pulses*	
1 whole pig's kidney (140g)	9mg	Average portion spinach	1.7mg
1 portion black pudding (75g)	15mg	Large portion cabbage	0.7mg
8oz/225g lean beef steak	6mg	Large portion peas	1.4mg
4oz/100g lean minced beef	2.7mg	225g can baked beans in	
2 thick slices corned beef	2.9mg	tomato sauce	3.2mg
Pate, low-fat slice on bread (40g)	2.5mg	120g cooked red lentils (3 tbsp)	2.9mg
1 chicken breast	0.65mg	120g cooked brown or green	
1 chicken quarter	2.0mg	lentils (3 tbsp)	4.2mg
1 small can tuna in brine	1.0mg	Average portion tofu (bean curd)	0.7mg
1 large fillet white fish	0.5mg		
6 cockles	6.2mg	*Nuts*	
6 mussels	3.2mg	25g bag cashew nuts	1.6mg
1 size 3 egg	1.1mg	1 tablespoon sesame seeds	1.1mg
Cereals		*Fruit*	
2 slices white bread	1.0mg	12 ready to eat dried apricots	3.4mg
2 slices wholemeal bread	1.9mg	6 dried dates	1.0mg
Breakfast cereals*		2 tablespoons raisins	0.8mg
Pasta, cooked av portion (7½ tbsp)	1.8mg		

* Many breakfast cereals are enriched with iron. Check the nutritional information panel on the box.

Increasing Iron Intake

The RNI for iron for women (aged 11–50 years) is 14.8mg a day and for adult men it is 8.7mg a day. (The RNI for women is higher to make up for iron losses during monthly periods.) Eating red meat, if appropriate, is the easiest way to ensure an adequate iron intake. Breakfast cereals that are fortified with iron are also a good choice, especially as they may be eaten very regularly in good amounts.

Vitamin C helps the absorption of iron, particularly from non-haem iron foods, so including a glass of orange or grapefruit juice with breakfast cereals, adding tomatoes and peppers to sandwiches and cooked dishes, and drinking squashes containing added vitamin C with meals can all help to boost intake. Strong tea and coffee should be drunk between meals rather than with them as the tannins present can reduce iron absorption. Absorption of iron from vegetables and cereals can be improved by eating a source of animal protein, such as red meat, at the same meal. Wholegrain breads and cereals are better choices than those with added bran as excessive bran intakes can reduce iron absorption.

Non-meat eaters should ensure that their diet contains some of the following on a daily basis:

- wholegrain cereals and flours (wheat, rye, millet, oatmeal);
- nuts (almonds, brazils, cashews, hazelnuts);
- dark green leafy vegetables (cabbage, watercress, spinach, broccoli, parsley);
- pulses (lima beans, soybeans, chickpeas, baked beans, lentils);
- eggs;
- dried fruit (apricots, prunes, raisins); and
- seeds (pumpkin, sesame, sunflower).

Miscellaneous items such as brewer's yeast, curry powder, textured vegetable protein, soya flour, black treacle, molasses, chocolate, cocoa and ginger can all make small but useful occasional contributions.

SALT

Many health professionals encourage a reduction in salt intake because of the possible link between regular high intakes and the development of high blood pressure. For runners, however, salt losses in sweat need to be replaced. Keeping intakes above this general public recommendation could benefit runners when sweat losses are high, provided that kidneys are healthy and overall fluid intake is good. The simplest way to increase salt intake when sweat losses have been high is to add it to meals at the table.

ANTIOXIDANTS

Regular exercise may have positive effects on the immune system but concerns have been raised that such benefits will be outweighed by the production of free radicals and oxidative stress, which occurs during exercise. These free radicals seem to be closely involved in exercise-induced tissue and cell damage. The rate of free-radical production may overwhelm the body's capacity to mop them up before they do too much damage. This is more likely to occur during prolonged aerobic exercise such as distance running. To protect against the harmful effects of oxidative stress, the body produces antioxidant compounds and enzymes. It also uses several dietary antioxidants including vitamins A (as the precursor beta-carotene), C and E, as well as zinc, selenium and phytochemicals.

Damage done by free radicals at the tissue and cellular level may be the cause of the muscle damage, soreness or inflammation that is often experienced after strenuous exercise. Runners who habitually have a low intake of fresh fruit and vegetables, or who are restricting intake to lose weight, may benefit from some supplementation. At the moment, it seems unlikely that supplementing with anything more than a simple multivitamin/mineral supplement, or a supplement containing the antioxidant nutrients in doses similar to the RDA, is needed. According to the International Olympic Committee Consensus Conference on Sports Nutrition (2003), there is a lack of convincing evidence that high doses of antioxidant vitamins, glutamine, zinc, probiotics and echinachea prevent exercise-induced immune impairment.

Evidence does suggest that those who exercise regularly are less prone to damage than those whose training is more erratic and haphazard. The runner following an intense, regular training programme may therefore benefit less from supplements than the individual who is running as and when time permits.

Supplementation aside, all athletes would benefit from having five portions of fruit and vegetables on a daily basis as these supply both antioxidant vitamins and phytochemicals.

FIVE A DAY: WHAT COUNTS AS A PORTION?

Large fruit (grapefruit, mango, melon, papaya and pineapple) – 1 large slice

Medium fruit (apple, avocado, banana, orange, peach, pear) – 1 whole fruit

Small fruit (apricot, clementine, fig, kiwi fruit, passion fruit, plum, satsuma, tangerine and tomato) – 2 whole fruits

Very small fruit (blackberries, blackcurrants, bilberries, cherries, cranberries, gooseberries, grapes, raspberries, strawberries) – 1 cupful

Fresh fruit salad, stewed or canned fruit – 3 tablespoons

Dried fruit (apricots, bananas, cranberries, currants, dates, figs, papaya, pineapple, raisins, sultanas) – 1 tablespoon

Fruit and vegetable juice (freshly squeezed or processed but not fruit drinks) – 1 medium glass (150ml). (Still counts as one portion regardless of how many glasses are drunk.)

Mixed salad vegetables (for example, celery, cucumber, lettuce, peppers, tomatoes) – 1 dessert bowlful

Vegetables (raw, cooked, frozen or canned) – 2 tablespoons

What does count?
Fresh, frozen, canned, 100 per cent juice and dried fruit and vegetables all count.

What does not count?
Potatoes, yam, cassava, nuts and seeds, coconut, marmalade, jam, fruit 'drinks' and squashes do not count.

INCREASING INTAKE OF ANTIOXIDANTS

Choose an assortment of colours to get a variety of phytochemicals, for example, lycopene in tomatoes.

Ready-chopped salads lose some of their nutrients. Boost content by adding another fresh vegetable.

Have a citrus fruit or drink every day.

Cook with onions and garlic.

Have tomatoes, raw, cooked or tinned, several times a week.

Snack on canned or dried fruits when favourite fresh fruits are out of season.

Add vegetables to canned soups.

Snack on raw vegetables and salsa.

Unfortunately, statistics show that young men and women are least likely to eat the recommended five portions a day. Older women are most likely to achieve the target.

ALCOHOL

Alcohol is not a significant source of fuel during exercise. Although the by-products formed when alcohol is broken down and released by the liver may find their way into muscles, they appear to be of little importance as a fuel source. The amount of oxygen needed to release energy from alcohol is greater than for an equivalent amount of carbohydrate or fat; if alcohol were to be used, it would be a very uneconomical process. In any case, the liver metabolizes alcohol far too slowly to make it a useful energy source. During prolonged exercise, alcohol interferes with glucose metabolism. When the liver metabolizes alcohol, the glucose output decreases, thereby increasing the risk of hypoglycaemia. Fuel starts to run out earlier, fatigue sets in and the running pace slows down. Alcohol ingestion may also impair body-temperature regulation during long runs in the cold.

Cardiovascular performance is not adversely affected if only one or two alcohol drinks have been consumed the night before, although a heavy night will probably impair performance next day mainly because of the hangover. A hangover is caused by alcohol toxicity, dehydration and the toxic effects of the congeners in some drinks. Depressed mood, headache and hypersensitivity to outside stimuli are common symptoms. As a result, a runner with a hangover may not feel like running and, if they decide to do it, they will almost certainly not run well or enjoy it. The major effect of alcohol intake on refuelling after running is indirect. Large intakes of alcohol are likely to compromise carbohydrate intake and prevent efficient glycogen storage.

Alcohol is a diuretic but in moderation it has little effect on the average person's state of fluid balance. If a runner is going to run again in the next twenty-four hours, alcohol intake should be limited to one or two units. Drinks with an alcohol content of less than 4 per cent (weak/light beers or lagers) can actually help to counter the effects of mild dehydration rather than make them worse, particularly if refuelling foods contain reasonable amounts of sodium.

The general consensus suggests an upper weekly limit of twenty-one units for men and fourteen units for women; drinks should be spread through the week; binge drinking should be avoided and there should be two or three alcohol-free days a week. A single measure of spirits or liqueur, a small glass of wine, sherry or fortified wine or half a pint of regular strength lager, beer or cider all represent one unit. A little alcohol, particularly red wine, may offer some protection against heart disease.

READING FOOD LABELS

Nutrition Information

Food labels can help a runner to make wise food choices, work out their own individual refuelling snacks and tot up daily carbohydrate intakes. Nutritional labelling is not compulsory, although most manufacturers and retailers do provide it voluntarily on the vast majority of products. If nutrition information is given, it has to be given in an order that is laid down by legislation. When minimum labelling is given, it must show the following:

- energy in kilojoules (kJ) or kilocalories (kcal);
- protein in grams (g);
- carbohydrate in grams (g);
- total fat in grams (g).

More detailed nutritional information can be given in the following format:

- energy (kJ/kcal);
- protein (g);
- carbohydrate (g),
  of which sugars (g);
- fat (g),
  of which saturates (g);
- fibre (g);
- sodium (g).

Some labels, particularly on breakfast cereal boxes, even indicate values for certain vitamins and minerals that have been added in the manufacturing process. Some labels also give the Official Government figures for Guideline Daily Amounts for calorie and fat intakes for average men (2,500kcal/95g fat) and average women (2,000kcal/70g fat). It must be emphasized that these figures are for the general population who, for the large part, do very little physical activity. They are not applicable to anybody who exercises regularly and particularly not to those training to run a marathon.

Dates

By law, food products must carry a 'best before' or a 'use by' date. The 'best before' date indicates the period during which the food keeps its specific properties, when stored correctly. In other words, if a product has expired its 'best before' date, it will still be safe to eat but the manufacturer no longer guarantees the taste, smell and appearance of the product. The 'use by' date is found on highly perishable products, which, from a microbiological point of view, are considered to pose a health risk if not eaten by that date. The manufacturer should also explain on the label how such products must be stored, for example, at or below a certain temperature.

RUNNING TIMES

Early Morning

For those who run early in the morning, breakfast may be a problem. Some people can eat breakfast and run soon after without any ill-effects. Others manage a small breakfast and have the bulk of the meal straight after training. (Breakfast cereal and toast – low in fat and high in carbohydrate – is ideal for refuelling.) Some people can run without any breakfast and still put in a good session, but others who skip breakfast will feel weak and light-headed during training.

Training is all about teaching the body to do things it has not been able to do before – including running faster or for longer. It is also possible to teach the body to get used to having breakfast and then running soon after.

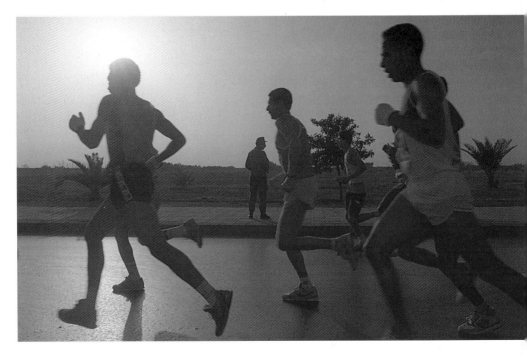

Running in the midday sun. (EMPICS)

Going from nothing to a large bowl of cereal and a pile of toast is likely to lead to disaster, but starting small and building up the intake gradually will not. On waking, use the bathroom, then make half a slice of toast and pour a small glass of fruit juice. Eat the mini-breakfast, change into training kit, warm up and stretch, then set off running. This gives the maximum time between eating breakfast and running, so any discomfort should be negligible. Another mini-breakfast can be eaten on returning from running, to start the refuelling process. With time, the amount eaten can be increased.

Early-morning runs should improve for having breakfast. As most marathons are run in the morning, getting in the breakfast habit can only be beneficial for the big event.

Lunchtime

Those who run in their lunch break should have a good high-carbohydrate breakfast and then have a mid-morning carbohydrate snack, ideally about two hours before they are due to start running. What is eaten will depend on circumstances but suitable snacks that can be

---

BREAKFAST SUGGESTIONS

Breakfast cereals with low-fat milk and dried or fresh fruit.

Muesli with fresh fruit and low-fat yoghurt.

Porridge cooked with milk and raisins.

Chopped fresh and/or dried fruit with low-fat yoghurt.

Toast, bread, muffins or bagels with low-fat spread and marmalade, honey or jam, Marmite or Vegemite, peanut butter or chocolate spread (omitting the low-fat spread), low-fat soft cheese and tomatoes.

Banana milk shake using low-fat milk.

Fruit smoothie.

Cooked breakfast

Baked beans on toast.

Grilled lean bacon sandwich.

Poached egg on toast.

Boiled egg with bread or toast.

Grilled tomatoes, lean grilled bacon, mushrooms and toast.

Omelettes stuffed with baked beans, mushrooms or tomatoes.

Potato cakes with tomatoes and mushrooms.

Pancakes with maple syrup.

Glass of fruit juice with any of the above.

PACKED LUNCH AND SNACK IDEAS

Sandwiches: ring the changes with the bread and filling combinations, and include some vegetables.

Fresh fruit, dried fruit, canned fruit, fruit and nuts.

Cereal bars, breakfast bars, cake bars, Jaffa Cakes, fig rolls and ginger snaps.

Fruit cake, parkin, gingerbread, fruit loaf, malt loaf, banana bread, Scotch pancakes, plain iced buns, scones and tea cakes.

Low-fat yoghurts and rice puddings, fromage frais, milk shakes and fruit smoothies.

Pretzels, rice cakes and Twiglets.

Fruit juice, squash, soft drinks, water or hot drinks.

eaten at work (without offence to others) include bananas, dried fruit, cereal bars, Jaffa Cakes, malt loaf, currant buns, scones and smoothies. Those with access to a kitchen can always have some toast and jam. For both lunchtime runners and those who run at other times of the day, it is a good idea to keep a bottle of water close at hand throughout the day so that fluid intake is constantly being topped up.

Time may be tight to run and have lunch, but some refuelling and rehydrating must be carried out. Refuelling after the run may be best achieved by preparing a packed meal at home and bringing it to work, so time will not be wasted queuing at sandwich bars or in work cafeterias or restaurants.

Evening

Runners may come home from work very hungry but with no time to eat before setting off for their run. Alternatively, they manage to run but then get back so hungry that they cannot wait to prepare a sensible meal and instead snack on all sorts while getting dinner ready. Runners should make sure they eat well throughout the day – no skipping breakfast, making lunch the main meal of the day if practical, having a mid-afternoon snack of fruit, cereal or energy bars, and so on – and keep up an impressive intake of fluids. There will be no need to eat a huge meal in the evening if a good, steady intake has been maintained through the day.

Ready meals can be a convenient option when time is short and there are just not enough minutes to prepare, cook and eat. Microwaveable 'healthy' options are the best choices, although some hungry runners may need two portions. Including a side salad, some bread, fruit and a glass of milk or a yoghurt will add up to a decent well-balanced meal.

It is a myth that eating close to bedtime causes weight increase. Eating a high-carbohydrate meal will put the fuel back into the muscles, not into the fat cells. Of course, a daily intake greater than the body needs, regardless of meal timings, will lead to an increase in body fat and body weight. At some time before bed, it is a good idea to think about what has been eaten during the day and spot if anything is missing. How much fruit has been

---

MAIN MEAL IDEAS

Shepherd's pie or cottage pie made with extra lean mince or Quorn or soya, peas and carrots.

Pasta with tomato sauce and tuna.

Chicken, lean beef, prawn stir-fry, tofu or Quorn pieces with vegetables and rice or noodles.

Grilled lean meat with mashed or boiled potatoes and vegetables.

Roast chicken or lean meat with jacket potato and vegetables.

Grilled fish fingers with mashed potatoes and vegetables.

Chicken, vegetable or lentil curry with rice.

Baked or grilled fish with jacket potatoes and vegetables.

Pasta with a lean Bolognese or Quorn/soya mince sauce and salad.

Rice with a lean beef, Quorn or soya mince chilli con carne and salad.

Rice with red kidney bean and vegetable sauce.

Macaroni cheese and grilled tomatoes.

Deep-pan pizza with lean ham and pineapple, tomatoes and sweetcorn.

Risotto with tuna, salmon pieces, lean ham or cooked chicken.

SUITABLE DESSERTS OR PUDDINGS (IF NECESSARY)

Fruit crumble with custard.

Milk puddings with jam or dried fruit.

Pancakes with maple syrup or golden syrup.

Baked apples with dried fruit and custard.

Instant whips with low-fat milk.

Sponge and custard.

Banana and custard or yoghurt.

Fruit in jelly with custard or yoghurt.

Yoghurt, fromage frais, Müllerice.

---

eaten? How much milk, yoghurt or cheese? Was carbohydrate intake sufficient? Any gaps can be plugged before bed by having a banana or some dried fruit, a glass of milk, or a couple of rounds of toast and honey. Nobody should go to bed hungry; instead, turn the day upside down and have a bowl of breakfast cereal and milk.

KEEPING A DIARY

Keeping a food diary of what, when and how much is eaten and drunk on a daily basis can help to identify possible problems when training is not going so well. This could be due to inadequate refuelling, forgetting water bottles on longer runs, missing breakfast regularly in exchange for more sleep, and many other reasons. A well-kept diary may alert a runner to a change in routine they were unaware of, such as dropping the mid-morning snack because of a change in their working situation.

WEIGHT LOSS

Many people take up running to lose weight. For many, just the extra calorie cost of running with some fine tuning to the balance of carbohydrate and fat in the diet will be all that is needed to achieve their goal. For some, a little more effort will be required on the diet side of the energy equation. With the additional benefit of regular running, cutting back by just 250–500kcal a day will, for most runners who genuinely need to lose weight, be enough to lose one to two pounds a week. The current diet should be checked for fat and alcohol content, as cutting back on these may be all that is needed to create the necessary deficit for the majority of people. Even when running to lose weight, refuelling after training remains a priority. It is false to assume that, having used up some calories in running, staying in deficit will encourage weight loss. In fact, running performance will suffer, with the result that fewer calories will be used up. *Fat* loss is the goal and not *weight* loss per se, so clothes that start to fit more loosely are a better indicator of success than a reading on the scales.

Slightly more emphasis should be placed on high-fibre foods, fresh fruit and vegetables, lean meat and low-GI foods in general. This will help to keep hunger at bay while still providing essential carbohydrate. Sports drinks should be used sensibly. Generally, they are not needed until runs are lasting an hour or more. It is still possible to overeat on healthy food so portion sizes should be checked, too. This can be achieved simply by using a smaller plate. It is also important to avoid going for long periods without food; it is much better to eat little and often. Although it is small, there is a calorie cost every time food is digested and absorbed (thermic effect of food).

Running is one of the most efficient ways to burn calories and covering distance rather than running faster helps to use up unwanted fat stores. It costs more in calories to move a heavier body so weight will come off faster initially. Running first thing in the morning also encourages weight loss because insulin levels are low and glucagon levels high. Insulin increases the uptake of glucose from the blood by the tissues and promotes synthesis of glycogen in the liver and muscles. It also promotes synthesis of fat. Glucagon has the opposite effect to insulin. It raises blood-glucose level, increases the rate of glycogen breakdown and promotes breakdown of fat. In other words, glucagon increases the availability of energy for exercise and insulin decreases it. As mileage really starts to increase, a diet of a higher energy value will be needed but by then the required fat (and weight) loss should have been achieved. With less dead weight to carry around, running should be an even better experience.

CHAPTER 3

Training Fluids

WATER

Water and the Body

Humans can survive for up to fifty days without food, yet only a few days without fluids. Roughly 60 per cent of a typical male's and 50 per cent of a typical female's body weight is made up of water. Approximately two-thirds

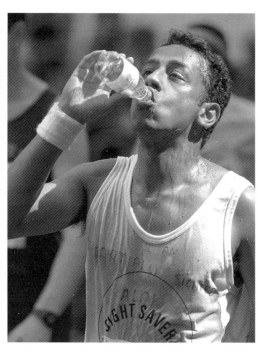

Drinking during the Flora London Marathon. (EMPICS)

of the water is found inside cells (intracellular fluid); the remainder is in the fluids outside the cells (extracellular fluid). Blood, lymph, cerebrospinal fluid and the fluid actually between the cells themselves make up the extracellular fluid. It is reasonable to expect such a ubiquitous fluid to have many functions in the body and this is precisely the case.

Requirements

It is generally agreed that healthy adults need between 2 and 3 litres of fluid each day. This is approximately equivalent to the amount that is lost every day. Training or racing in a hot environment, such as that experienced by

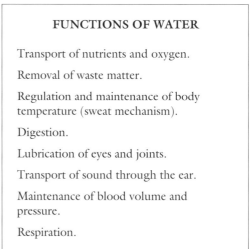

FUNCTIONS OF WATER

Transport of nutrients and oxygen.

Removal of waste matter.

Regulation and maintenance of body temperature (sweat mechanism).

Digestion.

Lubrication of eyes and joints.

Transport of sound through the ear.

Maintenance of blood volume and pressure.

Respiration.

DAILY WATER BALANCE

Daily water input		Daily water losses	
Food	1,000ml	Urine	1,250ml
Drinks	1,200ml	Faeces	100ml
Metabolism	350ml	Skin	850ml
		Lungs	350ml
Total	2,550ml	*Total*	2,550ml

Typical figures for a sedentary 70–75kg male living in a temperate climate.

On average, about 62 per cent of the daily fluid intake comes from drinks; milk, milk shakes and yoghurts contribute just over 10 per cent; bread and cereals 8 per cent; meat, fish, eggs and pulses 2 per cent; and fruit and vegetables 18 per cent. Alcohol in moderation has little impact on the average person's fluid balance, indeed, weak alcoholic drinks such as shandy or light beer can even be used to

WATER CONTENT OF SELECTED FOODS

Type of food	Water content (g per 100g edible portion)
Butter, margarine	15
Low-fat spread	53
Bananas	75
Carrots	90
Broccoli	91
Dried dates	14
Lettuce	95
Melon	92
Oranges	86
Peas	75
Tomatoes	93
Chips	52
Crisps, lower fat	1
Potatoes, boiled	80
Chicken	75
Eggs	75
Steak, lean, grilled	63
Peanuts, plain	6
White fish	82
Cheese	36
Milk	89
Yoghurt, fruit	76
Vegetable oil	Trace

(Data from Food Standards Agency (2002) McCance and Widdowson, *The Composition of Foods*, Sixth summary edition, Cambridge: Royal Society of Chemistry.)

athletes at the 2004 Olympic Games in Athens, raises daily fluid requirements to as much as 6 or 7 litres, or even more. Some of this is obviously provided by food intake but 4 or more litres will need to be supplied by drinks.

Unlike fat and carbohydrate, excess water cannot be stored for use at a later date. A regular fluid intake is therefore needed to keep the body well hydrated and all bodily functions dependent on water working well. Fluids are obviously vital for sustaining life, but there are a number of myths surrounding their use. The popular belief is that as many as eight 250ml glasses of water must be drunk a day for optimum health and well-being. There is, however, little evidence to support this claim. Many runners also believe that water is the best fluid to drink, even during a marathon. Again, there is plenty of evidence to show this is not true. Any drinks, with the possible exception of most alcoholic drinks, will contribute to overall fluid intake, including juices, tea, fruit and herbal teas, coffee, squashes and other soft drinks. Another surprise is that the contribution to overall fluid intake from food is only marginally smaller than that from fluid. This will be particularly true if the diet contains a healthy amount of fruit and vegetables.

quench thirst and counter the effects of dehydration rather than exacerbate them. Excessive amounts of alcohol do have a diuretic effect and dehydration is one of the causes of hangover symptoms.

Water Choices

People buy water for a variety of reasons, particularly because of a taste preference but also because of concerns about the quality of tap water. Water-borne diseases such as cholera or typhoid are now a thing of the past in the developed world, but many people still have concerns about possible contaminants in tap water, including lead, nitrates and hormones. In fact, the Water Quality Regulations (UK) imposes very strict standards that are far more stringent than those applied to bottled waters.

The most frequently stated reasons for not drinking tap water are the taste and smell. Some consumers particularly dislike the hint of chlorine that they can often detect; this is added to disinfect the water and prevent bacterial growth. A recent novel approach has been the introduction of Vivatap, a teabag-like sachet containing coral algae, shell, antioxidants and chitosan, which immediately removes all chlorine from tap water as well as adding useful minerals – at a fraction of the cost of bottled mineral water.

Mineral waters are subject to rigorous controls and the levels of minerals are carefully controlled. The source of water and mineral analysis must be printed on the label. Most of the minerals in the diet will still be derived from food rather than water. Perversely, even tap water can contain more naturally-occurring minerals essential for health than some mineral waters. Intakes of calcium and also magnesium in hard-water areas can help top up low dietary intakes, yet filtered water is often chosen instead of tap water precisely because of the amount of calcium in the water. Spring waters are not subject to the same regulations as mineral waters and the composition does not have to be the same, although brands do maintain consistency. Bottled waters often contain higher levels of harmless bacteria than ordinary tap water and, contrary to popular belief, do not necessarily contain lower nitrate levels. Legally, there is no upper limit on nitrate levels in natural mineral water, yet all other types of water, including tap water, have an upper limit of 50mg per litre. It is therefore always important to read the bottle label.

Jug filters can be used to get rid of the smell and taste of chlorine in tap water while point-of-use systems plumbed into the kitchen sink provide filtered water 'on tap'. Reverse osmosis and distillation are the most elaborate and expensive methods of supplying purified water and, although more or less all contaminants are removed, the process removes virtually all minerals, too. There are pros and cons for all types of water and, whatever the choice, the taste must appeal.

FLUIDS AND RUNNING

A deficit of only 1 or 2 per cent of body weight can affect performance and yet a runner may have no sensation of thirst and therefore no awareness of a need to take on board fluids. A 2 per cent loss in body weight can reduce aerobic capacity by up to 20 per cent and a 5 per cent loss by as much as 30 per cent. Indeed, a loss of as little as 1 per cent can have a marginal but nevertheless important effect on an individual's running performance. There is no point at which dehydration has no effect on performance and then suddenly does have an effect. Overall, dehydration hinders performance in terms of strength, speed, endurance, concentration and co-ordination.

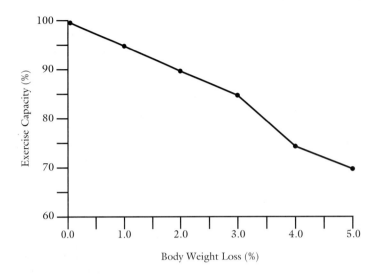

Effect of dehydration on exercise capacity.

SWEATING

Rate of Sweating

Sweat rate varies considerably between individuals even when running at the same pace, for the same length of time, in the same environmental conditions. Not only does the sweat rate vary, but the actual composition can vary enormously, too. The electrolyte concentration of sweat is lower than that of blood. This means that relatively more water than electrolytes is lost from the blood. Therefore,

dehydration due to sweat loss leads to an increase in the concentration of blood electrolytes. However, this is only the case when water is not ingested to compensate for fluid loss. Large sweat losses and compensation by plain water alone can induce a low blood-sodium level (hyponatraemia).

Variations in Sweat Rate

Exercise Intensity

As exercise intensity increases, so does the sweat rate. When exercise intensity increases to high levels (>75 per cent VO_2max), the rate at which ingested fluid can be digested and absorbed by the stomach and intestines, and ultimately reach the bloodstream, is reduced. Sweat losses at 10km pace will therefore be greater than at marathon pace, assuming environmental conditions are the same. However, total sweat losses will be greater in the marathon because of the duration of the event. Faster runners produce more heat and sweat more but drink less than slower runners

---

INDIVIDUAL VARIATIONS IN SWEAT COMPOSITION	
Volume	500ml–3 litres per hour
Sodium (Na)	20–80mmol per litre
Chloride (Cl)	20–60mmol per litre
Potassium (K)	4–8mmol per litre
Calcium (Ca)	0–1mmol per litre
Magnesium (Mg)	<0.2mmol per litre

because they avoid slowing down in order to take a drink.

Environmental Temperature

Sweat losses are greater at higher ambient temperatures, as the body's usual methods of getting rid of heat (conduction, convection and radiation) are unable to cope. In cool conditions, sweating usually begins about seven minutes after exercise has started.

Humidity

In a humid environment the atmosphere contains more moisture than usual and this reduces the effectiveness of the sweat mechanism to cool the body down. It is actually the evaporation of sweat from the skin that has a cooling effect on the skin and, ultimately, on the rest of the body. If the atmosphere is very moist, sweat drips rather than evaporates from the skin and cooling of the skin is therefore minimal. This

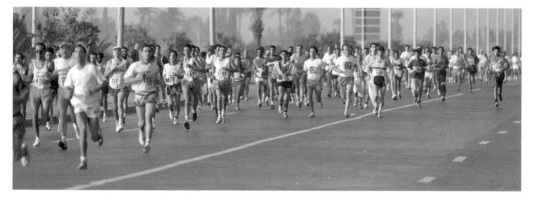

The Marrakesh Marathon, Morocco. (EMPICS)

APPROXIMATE FLUID LOSSES DURING RUNNING IN DIFFERENT CONDITIONS

Distance	Sex	Intensity	Sweat rate	Percentage body weight loss (%)	Ambient temp. (°C)	Relative humidity
10km	f	12.8km/h	1.49kg/h	1.8	19–24	–
10km	m	14.6km/h	1.83kg/h	1.8	19–24	–
42.2km	–	9.3–15.5km/h	1.1kg/h	3.7	21–26	50–60
42.2km	f	9–12km/h	0.54kg/h	2.6	6–24	45–85
42.2km	m	9–12km/h	0.81kg/h	3.4	7	45–85
42.2km	m	8.7–16.1km/h	0.96kg/h	2.9	10–12	73
42.2km	m	15.9km/h	1.52kg/h	6.0	20	37

Adapted from Rehrer, N.J. and Burke, L.M. (1996), *Aust J Nutr Diet* 1996; 53 (4 Suppl.): S13–S16.

results in fluid loss but minimal regulation of body temperature.

Body Surface Area

A larger body surface has a greater evaporative, and therefore cooling, capacity. Therefore the larger the body surface area, the greater the sweat loss.

Gender Differences

Females generally have a smaller plasma volume and a lower percentage of body water than most males. Therefore, if a male and female runner were losing sweat at the same rate, the female runner would be losing a greater proportion of her body water and plasma volume. Females, however, tend to sweat less than males in the same conditions.

Hydration Status

As dehydration intensifies and plasma volume drops, sweat rate is reduced and regulation of body temperature becomes less and less well controlled. In other words, dehydration reduces the body's ability to meet the thermal stress of exercise.

Acclimatization

Training in the heat helps runners to adapt by enabling the body to sweat more and initiate sweating earlier. This adaptation or improved tolerance to running in a hot environment is known as heat acclimatization. It can take up to ten days to become completely acclimatized, although the major effects will have kicked in after a week. Once acclimatized, runners must continue to take fluid on board earlier and in greater amounts than normal. The same advice would apply to runners continuing their training while holidaying in a hot country.

Clothing

Light, loose clothing allows sweat to evaporate from the body and will therefore not hinder temperature regulation of the body.

Individuality

Of course, some runners do just sweat more than others.

Fancy Dress

Many marathon runners, particularly those raising money for charity, wear fancy dress on the day. Wearing hats, special T-shirts or carrying small placards are all ways of attracting attention which do not hinder running or endanger health. On the other hand, runners who choose

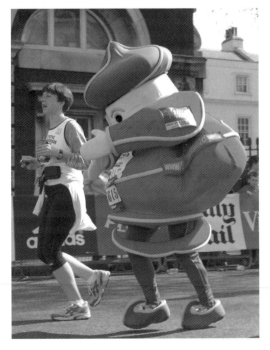

Runner in fancy dress at the Flora London Marathon 2003. (EMPICS)

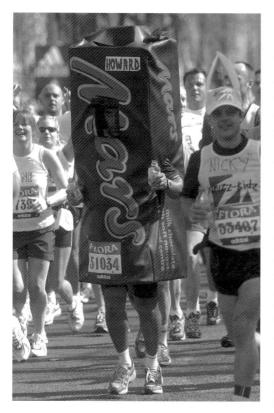

Runner in fancy dress with fluids at the
Flora London Marathon 2003. (EMPICS)

those losses. Only general guidelines can be given, and runners must establish their own individual fluid strategies. The optimum frequency, volume and composition of drinks used, before, during and after running will vary widely, depending on the various factors. Runners must use training runs and less important races to identify what strategy works best for them and which suitable drinks are the most palatable and acceptable.

DEHYDRATION

Dehydration decreases plasma volume, which causes an increase in heart rate and a decrease in stroke volume. It also causes an increase in serum osmolality, which reduces blood flow to the skin. The ability of the body to dissipate body heat as running continues is impaired, the core body temperature starts to increase at a faster rate and considerable strain is placed on the cardiovascular system. For every extra litre of sweat loss that is not replaced by fluid intake, the rectal temperature increases by 0.3°C, cardiac output falls by 1 litre per minute, heart rate increases by eight beats per minute, and the perceived rate of exertion increases rapidly. It is hardly surprising that running performance suffers.

The body cannot be trained to get used to dehydration. After all, sweating is one of the body's safety mechanisms, its way of protecting a rise in core body temperature. Unfortunately, thirst is not a very good indicator of dehydration. A significant level of dehydration can occur before a runner feels any desire to drink. If dehydration is allowed to persist, a runner can ultimately become disorientated, experience heat flushes, feel abnormally chilly, or vomit. In very extreme cases, runners can develop heat stroke, a serious condition that requires immediate medical attention (*see* Chapter 6).

to wear fancy dress that leaves little or no skin uncovered will be putting themselves at risk of overheating. This will be exacerbated if the attire prevents the runner from drinking during the entire race. Those who choose to draw attention to themselves should do so in a way that is not going to put them at risk of serious dehydration.

Replacing Losses that Occur through Sweating

With so many variables, it is impossible to predict fluid losses accurately and very difficult to calculate the fluid intake needed to replace

COMMON SIGNS AND SYMPTOMS ASSOCIATED WITH DEHYDRATION

Thirst	Dizziness	Loss of mental alertness
Irritability	Muscle cramp	Head or neck heat sensations
Headache	Fatigue	Loss of performance
Weakness	Nausea	
Light-headedness	Vomiting	

NOTE: by no means all these signs and symptoms are likely to be exhibited by an individual.

FLUID REPLACEMENT

Thirst

Thirst is a learned behaviour. Young children will demand a drink, take a sip and then leave the rest. Adults tend to wait to develop a thirst and then drink the whole drink. Even so, under normal resting conditions, thirst is an adequate stimulus for fluid replacement, as shown by the maintenance of water balance on a day-to-day basis in healthy, hydrated adults. However, the thirst mechanism is a relatively insensitive one and involuntary dehydration or an inability to match fluid intake to fluid loss is not uncommon during exercise, particularly when undertaken in warm/hot conditions. Runners exercising in the heat do not voluntarily replace all the fluid they lose through sweating. The thirst mechanism becomes apparent only when the body senses either a decrease in body water or an increase in sodium concentration (usually sensed by the brain cells). The sensation of thirst is therefore only experienced when the body becomes stressed by a significant loss of fluid and should therefore not be relied on as the stimulus to begin drinking during training or a race.

All runners have to train their body to get used to increasing the amount of fluid they drink in the same way that they train their body to do an increased mileage. Novice runners rarely replace sweat losses during exercise and all runners rarely replace sweat losses after exercise.

Cessation of Drinking

The reasons why people stop drinking are poorly understood. In a recent experiment, subjects were deprived of fluids for twenty-four hours. On rehydrating, they drank 65 per cent of their fluid consumption within two and a half minutes. The subsequent decrease in rate of fluid intake happened long before there was any noticeable change in the blood that was perfusing the brain. Most of the ingested fluid was still in the stomach or intestines. Plasma osmolality did not start to fall for another ten minutes. It seems that there may be volume receptors as well as osmoreceptors (cells that are sensitive to changes in osmotic pressure) in the mouth, throat, stomach and probably also the small intestine itself. These communicate with the brain to indicate how much fluid has been drunk. The receptors even give some information about the nature of the fluid; in the experiment, some drinks appeared to be much more thirst-quenching than others.

The Mechanics of Fluid Replacement

It is vital to get fluids into the body as quickly as possible. The potential hold-ups in achieving this are the speed at which fluid leaves the stomach and how quickly it is absorbed across the wall of the small intestine, passes into the circulation and, ultimately, into the muscle cells. A variety of factors affect stomach emptying. For instance, there is rapid emptying from the stomach initially but the rate slows as the volume decreases. Keeping the volume high is therefore a good strategy for rapid emptying. On the other hand, hypertonic solutions, high caloric density, a high fat content, acidity, a VO_2max greater than 75 per cent and dehydration itself all tend to slow down stomach emptying. The type of carbohydrate and the particular exercise undertaken do not appear to affect stomach-emptying time.

In the small intestine, the presence of glucose stimulates sodium uptake from the small intestine and this greatly increases fluid absorption. The active transport of glucose and sodium creates an osmotic gradient, which draws water across the gut wall. Other carbohydrates, such as sucrose or glucose polymers, can be substituted for glucose without impairing glucose or water uptake.

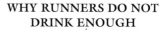

WHY RUNNERS DO NOT DRINK ENOUGH

Poor understanding of the need to maintain hydration.

Moistening of the mouth leads to a physiological inhibition of thirst.

Fear of stomach discomfort.

Fear of needing to urinate during a race restricts fluid intake prior to the race.

Flavour, taste, mouth-feel and temperature of the drink can all affect the amount that is drunk.

Not enough access to fluids, especially in training; difficulty in taking enough on long runs. (Problems are usually less in races, especially marathons.)

Avoidance of sports drinks because of their energy (calorie) value.

Forgetfulness.

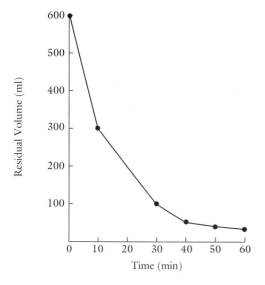

Speed of gastric emptying.

Sports Drinks

Sports drinks are formulated to enhance hydration and optimize performance. Some of the ingredients used in these drinks are based on sound science, others are a necessary part of the manufacturing process or are added to provide a stable, palatable drink with a reasonable shelf life. Additional ingredients may be included; these may give a commercial edge but there is usually less scientific or technical justification for their presence.

Carbohydrate

During exercise, the body uses 30–60g of carbohydrate every hour. If the onset of fatigue due to insufficient glycogen stores is to be delayed as long as possible, carbohydrate must be replaced regularly during exercise. Carbohydrate and water are rapidly absorbed from the small intestine when the concentration of carbohydrate is less than 10 per cent. As carbohydrate concentration increases above 10 per cent, absorption slows down. Glucose, sucrose and glucose polymers are the best forms of carbohydrate, although small amounts (2 to 3 per cent) of fructose can be used to improve the flavour and to supply a different form of carbohydrate. Fluid appears to be absorbed more quickly from the intestine if both glucose and fructose are present, compared with the presence of glucose alone. However, larger amounts of fructose may play a part in actually decreasing rates of absorption and oxidation. Large amounts of fructose may also cause gastrointestinal upsets. Replacing glucose with glucose polymers may help speed up stomach emptying, though the effect is only small if the total carbohydrate concentration is less than 10 per cent.

Isotonic – What Does It Mean?

An isotonic drink contains approximately the same number of molecules in solution as body fluids. They usually provide between 5 and 8 per cent carbohydrate – a concentration that does not compromise the delivery of fluid. Hypotonic drinks contain fewer molecules in solution than body fluids. Their lower osmolality promotes water uptake but invariably supplies less carbohydrate. Hypertonic drinks contain more molecules in solution than body fluids. They contain a greater concentration of carbohydrate and, though they deliver more energy, stomach emptying is slower and fluid replacement less effective.

Fatigue is invariably caused by depletion of glycogen stores and/or by dehydration. In the ideal situation, the type of drink used during exercise should reflect this. Rehydration will be the priority for marathon runners and therefore an isotonic drink containing no more than 8 per cent carbohydrate will be the best choice for the majority of runners. Fluid replacement must always take priority over provision of energy. This is because, although dehydration will affect performance, severe dehydration has health implications and in extreme cases can be life-threatening. Inadequate fuel supplies will only result in early fatigue.

Electrolytes

Sodium stimulates the absorption of both carbohydrate and water in the small intestine as the active co-transport of glucose and sodium creates an osmotic gradient that encourages net water absorption. The presence of sodium also encourages the desire to drink. Replacing sweat losses with plain water post-exercise can lead to a dilution of the blood if volumes are big enough. The consequent fall in plasma osmolality and sodium concentration reduces the drive to drink and stimulates urine output. Most sports drinks contain 10–25mmol sodium per litre. Higher levels of sodium encourage better fluid retention during rehydration. However, such levels are not as palatable, which could lead to an overall reduction in fluid intake. The level of sodium in most sports drinks is therefore a compromise between taste and physiological requirement.

The concentration of other electrolytes in sweat, such as potassium, calcium and magnesium, is low compared with sodium and chloride. There do not appear to be any data to suggest that these electrolytes need to be included in a sports drink designed for use before, during and immediately after exercise. Any losses after exercise will be made up by normal food intake. Having said that, most sports drinks do contain other electrolytes besides sodium, often in concentrations similar to those estimated to be present in sweat. Though unnecessary there do not appear to be any adverse effects of their presence. Such drinks are used widely and to date no reports of any problems have been published.

Other Ingredients

Some sports drinks contain added vitamins, minerals, protein and herbs. At the moment there is little evidence to suggest that these are of any benefit. A few products are carbonated and, although there is some evidence that gastric emptying is hastened if drinks are carbonated, such drinks, particularly the more heavily carbonated ones, are likely to cause gastrointestinal distress. Even mildly carbonated drinks can make a runner feel full and the negative aspect of this could well be a reduction in overall fluid intake.

Which Sports Drink?

A sports drink must contain carbohydrate, sodium and water; be hypotonic or isotonic; palatable and easy to use. Concentration of these ingredients must be such that they rehydrate the body fast and effectively while providing extra energy to top up the decreasing limited stores of carbohydrate. Using a sports drink before, during and after training can also help to minimize the risk of picking up an infection (*see* Chapter 1). Although taste will largely dictate which sports drink a runner chooses, it is wise to find out early on in training whether there is an official marathon sports drink. If there is, it should be used in training and certainly on longer runs prior to the race itself.

Some runners find the flavour and strength of sports drinks too intense, particularly when they need to drink large volumes. The practice of diluting these drinks with water may improve their palatability but it also dilutes the sodium concentration and reduces the efficiency of the formulation. Other runners are concerned about the energy or calorie

---

RECIPES FOR HOME-MADE SPORTS DRINKS

50–70g glucose or sucrose (ordinary sugar)
1 large pinch of salt (1.0–1.5g or one-fifth of a teaspoon)

Dissolve the sugar and salt in a little warm water. Flavour with low-sugar or low-calorie squash (not regular, as this will upset the balance of carbohydrate). Top up to a litre with water. Mix together, cover and keep chilled in the fridge.

500ml unsweetened fruit juice (for example, orange, pineapple or grapefruit)
500ml water
1 large pinch of salt (1.0–1.5g or one-fifth of a teaspoon)

Dissolve the salt in a little of the water, which has been warmed. Add the fruit juice and remaining water (not warmed). Mix together, cover and keep chilled in the fridge.

200ml squash (any flavour but not low-sugar or no-added-sugar varieties)
1 large pinch of salt (1.0–1.5g or one-fifth of a teaspoon)

Dissolve the salt in a little warm water. Add the squash and then make up to 1 litre with cool water. Mix together, cover and keep chilled in the fridge.

Make up a new batch of drink every day. Throw away any unused drink after twenty-four hours. Keep water bottles very clean as sugary drinks attract bugs and other nasty things. This is important at all times and especially during warm weather.

value of sports drinks, worrying that drinking large quantities will cause them to gain weight. This, of course, will only happen if their total energy intake is consistently greater than their energy expenditure. In this situation, runners should modify their eating habits to compensate for the additional carbohydrate supplied by the drinks, rather than choosing water as their hydration fluid. As 1 litre of a typical sports drink provides 50–70g carbohydrate (200–280kcal), most runners find that using a sports drink before, during and after training is beneficial not only to their fluid strategy but also to meeting their daily carbohydrate requirements.

Some runners prefer to make their own home-made isotonic drink rather than use commercial products. This may well be practical on training runs but could present problems when running in a half or full marathon race, where a commercial sports drink and water are usually provided. Sound advice is never to do something in a race that has not already been tried and tested in training and this would without doubt apply to use of an unfamiliar drink. Equally, drinking water during a race when a home-made drink has been used in training is not advisable either. Home-made sports drinks can be made using regular squashes and juices but both need careful dilution and addition of sodium in the form of ordinary table salt. This is because most fruit juices have a carbohydrate content of 10 per cent and negligible sodium content, and a squash made up to regular strength will also contain a similar amount of carbohydrate and negligible sodium.

ALTERNATIVE DRINKS

Runners should consume a range of drinks, including water (tap, bottled, fizzy or still), fruit juice, soft drinks, teas and coffees, throughout the day. Diet soft drinks including squashes and canned drinks may be appropriate, particularly for those who have taken up running specifically to help them lose weight. Coffee, tea and some soft drinks such as colas contain caffeine, which, in one large dose of 300mg or above, acts as a diuretic and so stimulates urine production. Increased urine production also occurs when caffeine is reintroduced into the diet after a number of days without any caffeine-containing drinks. In the past, the advice has been to encourage a reduction in intake or a switch to decaffeinated varieties. A single dose of 300mg is equivalent to the total amount in five to eight cups of tea, five to six cans of caffeine-containing carbonated soft drinks, or three to five cups of coffee. Single caffeine doses at the levels found in commonly consumed beverages have little or no diuretic effect. It also seems that regular drinkers of caffeine-containing drinks adapt to the caffeine intake and that the diuretic effects become even less apparent. Still, as with food, it is best to include a variety each day.

Water as an Alternative?

Before, during and immediately after longer training runs and races, a sports drink (commercial or home-made) will, in most cases, be the most appropriate drink. Certainly, the benefits of a sports drink over water will increase as mileage increases.

As water is not absorbed as quickly as a sports drink it is better used for low-intensity exercise only, when sweat losses will be negligible, or for short-duration exercise sessions lasting no more than forty-five minutes (for example, a 10km race). As carbohydrate stores will not be limited and sweat losses not enough to have a detrimental effect on running performance or health, there is really no need to drink anything. For many runners, the pace of a 10km race will make it hard to take on board fluids anyway.

Water can also be used in combination with a sports drink for variety, but in long runs sports drinks should always be the first choice. Research carried out at the Australian Institute of Sport in 1999 showed that flavoured drinks achieved a better fluid balance when compared with water. Even those athletes who said they preferred to drink water during exercise actually had a better fluid intake when encouraged and given the opportunity to drink a flavoured drink during exercise. The poor fluid intake with water is possibly because the thirst signals are suppressed before fluid losses have been replaced, the lack of flavouring is less of stimulus for intake and the lack of sodium reduces the osmotic drive to drink. Those who just drink water often only take enough to refresh themselves but not enough to maintain fluid balance or at least minimize dehydration. Runners who prefer to drink water must learn to drink 'beyond merely feeling refreshed'.

The high-calorie content of sports drinks is often perceived negatively, particularly by females, yet in long runs a sports drink can help a runner maintain running speed by topping up the flagging stores of muscle glycogen. Replacing sweat losses with plain water can even, in extreme cases, lead to hyponatraemia (*see* page 82).

Sports Water

Sports waters are hypotonic drinks, often made from purified water, with a lower carbohydrate content than sports drinks. Some contain added vitamins, minerals and electrolytes. They tend to have a lighter flavour than sports drinks, to counter the criticism that some sports drinks are too highly flavoured. Having a lower calorie content makes these drinks ideal for less intense training sessions when depleting carbohydrate stores are not an issue. In lower-intensity sessions, where sweat losses are low, sports waters will also be suitable but they are not the best choice when rapid rehydration is necessary. Some sports waters contain extra B vitamins and, although many of these are needed in energy release, there is no evidence to indicate that extra vitamins in these drinks will benefit or aid performance.

Oxygenated water is another product that has hit the market in recent years, with claims that it allows more oxygen to be delivered to the body and so enhances performance. It is questionable how much 'extra' oxygen is present by the time it is drunk, as most of the drinks are sold in plastic bottles, which are permeable to oxygen. Physiologically, it is not possible for oxygenated water to raise the level of oxygen in the blood or muscles, so the benefit of these drinks has to be questioned. However, on-going research is being undertaken in both Great Britain and the USA and there are early indications that some improvements in performance and recovery do occur, although the mechanisms for these improvements are as yet unclear.

Stimulant or Energy Drinks

These drinks are being marketed as boosting performance. A comparison with sports drinks shows that energy drinks are more likely to have a negative effect on performance if used before, during or after running. The main ingredients found in them are carbohydrate, vitamins, minerals, herbs and caffeine. Some also contain added amino acids. Their carbohydrate content is usually between 10 and 12 per cent, which is similar to soft drinks and higher than sports drinks. Sugar-free varieties have recently been introduced on to the market and these have negligible or very low levels of carbohydrate.

At the higher level of carbohydrate, rapid fluid absorption will be compromised, leading to an increased risk of dehydration. Sodium levels are not always declared so there may be no way of knowing how much they contain. Sports drinks, on the other hand, are formulated with special attention to sodium levels, so that the optimum level is achieved without compromising on taste. Energy drinks tend to be carbonated whereas sports drinks are still. Some energy drinks contain other substances, such as glucuronolactone, taurine and inositol, but there is no evidence that these substances afford any benefit to runners or enhance sports performance in general. As a result there has been a move to get manufacturers to put a clear statement on labels of such products stating that they are unsuitable hydration agents for use in sport and during exercise.

DRINK TEMPERATURE

In warm conditions, most runners prefer chilled drinks although some do enjoy drinks as cold as 5–10°C. Although runners appear to drink greater volumes of a cool drink compared with a warm drink, the actual temperature of the drink does not seem to be important physiologically. Whether drinks are chilled or at room temperature, they will quickly reach body temperature in the stomach. Tolerance to cold drinks is a very individual thing and, indeed, they can cause gastrointestinal upsets in some people. Temperature does not appear to influence stomach emptying in any way. A warm drink will not compromise the rehydration process, and could lift the spirits of a cold and tired individual returning from a run in wintry conditions.

ESTIMATING HYDRATION STATUS

Runners must work out their own fluid requirements rather than just applying general guidelines. Two runners of the same height and weight running together at the same speed for the same length of time will not necessarily sweat at the same rate. Runners who know approximately how much sweat they are likely to lose during runs of varying duration and intensity, and in different weather conditions, will be able to estimate how much they need to drink in order to minimize dehydration.

There are a few simple but excellent ways to assess hydration status: keeping a daily check on body weight, estimating fluid losses during training runs, and remaining alert to any changes in urinating habits. By weighing at the start of the day without clothing, using a reliable set of scales that ideally weigh to the nearest 100g, before breakfast but after a successful visit to the lavatory, a runner can track any progressive dehydration as the days go by. If a runner is well hydrated, body weight will remain relatively stable, varying by less than 0.5kg a day. A reduction in weight of more than 0.5kg from one day to the next is likely to be because body fluid levels have dropped – unless of course the runner is trying to lose weight by eating less.

Again using reliable scales, runners can weigh before and after running. Acute changes in weight will be due almost totally to loss of body water through sweating, as respiratory losses and depletion of glycogen stores will be relatively small. Weighing should be done without clothing and all traces of sweat should be removed by a brisk towel-down before stepping on to the scales. The aim is to make the weighing conditions before and after the run as close to identical as possible. Fluids (and food if applicable) consumed during the run must be noted and taken into account. Visits to the lavatory should be made before the pre-run weighing and after the post-run weighing – hopefully, there will not be any such losses during the actual run!

Sweat losses will continue for some time after the run and there are likely to be some

---

AN EXAMPLE OF HOW TO ESTIMATE SWEAT LOSS

Weight before running	60kg
Weight after running	58.5kg
Weight of fluid (and food) consumed during run	1kg (equivalent to 1ltr)
Duration of run	2 hours

Total sweat loss = 60 − 58.5 + 1 = 2.5kg

$$\text{Sweat rate} = \frac{2.5}{2} = 1.25 \text{ litres per hour}$$

---

urine losses even when a runner is dehydrated. This is because waste products still need to be eliminated from the body. As a result, runners are advised to drink 1.5 litres of fluid for every 1kg loss in weight, to ensure they hydrate fully. Calculating sweat losses during runs of different duration and in different weather conditions can help a runner to assess how much fluid should be drunk on future similar training runs. This can be invaluable if the weather suddenly becomes much warmer in the days leading up to and including the marathon itself. This method does not give any information about the hydration status of a runner at the beginning of the run, however.

As dehydration develops, urine colour darkens, and volume and frequency of urinating both decrease. The 'pee' test is therefore a simple way of detecting the level of hydration or dehydration. A well-hydrated person will frequently pass urine that is pale in colour (particularly as it gets later in the day), and in reasonable amounts. Infrequent, small volumes of dark urine are a warning sign of dehydration. Regular use of multivitamin supplements can make urine yellower in colour. This should then be considered the baseline colour and any further darkening from this could indicate dehydration. Other factors may affect the colour including certain foods (beetroot), medication and illness. Laminated credit-card-sized pee charts and A4 posters can be bought from Dietitians in Sport and Exercise Nutrition (*see* Appendix I for address). The chart gives eight graded colours, from very pale, almost colourless, to a rich brown colour.

Urinating a good volume between four and eight times in a twenty-four-hour period is normal. The actual number is determined by the amount of time someone is willing to 'hold on for'. Some people rush to the lavatory at the slightest urge while others wait as long as possible. The latter is the healthier option, as it allows the bladder to fill up properly. Women get the first desire to pass urine when the bladder contains about 200ml and need to empty it when 400–500ml has been collected. Because of the difference in anatomy, men

---

HYDRATION STATUS – GENERAL GUIDELINES OF INDICES

	Percentage body weight change	Urine colour
Well-hydrated	+1 to −1%	1 or 2
Minimal dehydration	−1 to −3%	3 or 4
Significant dehydration	−3 to −5%	5 or 6
Serious dehydration	>5%	>6

WHAT IS A 2 PER CENT BODY LOSS?

Pre-exercise body weight		Weight loss after exercise equivalent to 2 per cent of body weight	
kg	*lb*	*kg*	*lb*
50	110	1.0	2.2
60	132	1.2	2.6
70	154	1.4	3.0
80	176	1.6	3.5
90	198	1.8	4.0
100	220	2.0	4.4

tend to go longer before they need to urinate. Urinating every two to four hours is probably a reasonable sign that sufficient fluids are being consumed.

HOW MUCH TO DRINK?

It is clear (*see* also Chapter 4) that fluid requirements are a very individual thing and that even leading authorities do not agree about fluid

GENERAL FLUID REPLACEMENT GUIDELINES

400–600ml two hours before running, thus allowing time to excrete excess.

150–300ml in the 10 to 20 minutes before starting running, for example, during the warm-up (5–8ml per kg body weight).

150–250ml every 15 to 20 minutes (3–4ml per kg body weight). Runners must feel comfortable and should not be forcing fluids down. However, in most situations no more than 225ml of fluid every 20 minutes should be sufficient.

replacement guidelines. Advice to runners must be to drink to meet their own individual needs and to be aware that general guidelines are just that – guidelines.

Fluid intake should be increased slowly in the same way that mileage is increased gradually. Using a stopwatch or alarm can be helpful in reminding cautious or forgetful drinkers to use their water bottle. It takes no more than ten to twenty minutes for fluids to travel from the gut to the skin for sweating, hence the need to start drinking sooner rather than later. Thirst is an unreliable indicator of fluid requirements. Runners need to drink fluids before the stimulation of the thirst mechanism kicks in. Waiting until that point will invariably be too late to be of maximum benefit.

As training runs become longer it will probably be impossible to carry sufficient fluids to meet requirements. It may be necessary to arrange drinks along the route, to devise a run that laps around home, where empty bottles can be exchanged for full ones, or to encourage a minder to cycle alongside with supplies. A variety of bottles and systems can be tried and tested. Initially, on shorter runs, a simple running flask or bottle will be sufficient. 'Doughnut'-shaped ones do not hold a large volume, but are easy to grip and it is possible

THE NEED FOR SODIUM

Where sweat losses are high, the total sodium loss can be very high, too. Actual sodium losses will be very variable depending on the duration of the run, sweat rate and sodium content of the sweat. Five litres of sweat with a sodium concentration of 50mmol per litre is equivalent to a salt loss of nearly 15g. Making a moderate increase in dietary salt intake will help to restore euhydration (normal hydration) but will be unlikely to have any detrimental effects on health, as long as enough fluid is drunk and kidneys are functioning normally. Any excess sodium will be lost in the urine as the kidneys restore equilibrium. Salt tablets should be avoided, as they can irritate the gut and cause diarrhoea and vomiting. It is also quite likely that insufficient water will be taken with the tablets. Instead, salt should be added to food and a sports drink used before, during and after longer training runs and races.

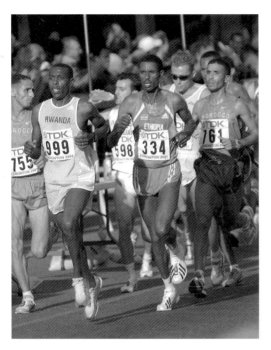

Leading runners at the IAAF World Championships Marathon, Edmonton. (EMPICS)

KEEPING HYDRATED

It is all too easy to concentrate on fluid intake around running and then forget about the overall daily fluid intake. Runners should aim for a regular fluid intake, using specific key points in the day to take on board fluids, for example, on waking, with meals, on arriving at work, mid-morning and mid-afternoon, getting home from work and bedtime. Using a large rather than a small cup can considerably increase the volume of fluid taken, particularly when added up over the day at work. Those who work in an air-conditioned environment for much of the day will need to compensate for greater fluid losses than those who do not. Including plenty of fruit and some milk in the daily diet will not only contribute to fluid intake but also push up intake of vital nutrients.

to run with one in each hand. A bottle belt worn around the waist allows empty bottles to be exchanged for full ones relatively easily. The 'camelbak' system is carried like a rucksack but is not refillable on the move.

Whatever system is used, scrupulous hygiene of the bottles and tubes is essential, particularly if a sports drink is used. Their formula makes them nutritionally appealing to fast-growing bacteria and provides a welcome breeding ground for them. Water bottles should never be shared with anybody else. Bottles should be washed thoroughly after every use with hot, soapy water, air-dried, and stored with lids off. Bottles should not be used for more than one day without being washed. Once or twice a week, bottles should be properly sterilized with a baby-bottle sterilizing fluid or denture-sterilizing tablets.

81

CARE OF TEETH

Runners are at risk of developing dental caries and dental erosion because of their higher intake of sugars and the use of sports drinks. Caries is caused by dental plaque (a thin layer of bacteria), which sticks to the teeth and breaks down sugars into acids, which then attack the teeth. Dental erosion does not involve bacteria but is the result of teeth being exposed to acidic foods and drinks. Both gastro-oesophageal reflux disease and eating disorders increase the risk of erosion, self-induced vomiting being the cause in the case of the latter. The main sources of acid in the diet are fruits (particularly citrus fruits), fruit juices, fruit-based and fizzy soft drinks, pickled foods or foods containing vinegar, and sports drinks.

Sports drinks should not be avoided because of the risk of developing dental erosion. Instead, great care should be taken to ensure the risks of erosion and decay are minimized as much as possible. Sports drinks should be drunk quickly, avoiding any sipping, holding or swishing of the fluid in the mouth. Where possible, cool drinks should be used, as this can help to reduce erosion. For at least an hour after using a sports drink (or any other acidic drink or food), brushing teeth should be avoided, but the mouth can be rinsed with a mouthwash. Sports drinks should be used only before, during and after running and intake of other acidic drinks during the day should be limited.

Sugar-free chewing gum is tooth-friendly. It clears away food debris and increases saliva production, which, being alkaline, helps to neutralize the acid. Gum should only be used after running; it should never be chewed while running, or indeed during any form of exercise, because of the risk of choking. Once teeth have been cleaned at bedtime, nothing more should be eaten or drunk, apart from water. This is because the flow of saliva falls during sleep. Finally, flossing and brushing with de-sensitizing fluoride toothpaste should be undertaken twice a day. Regular check-ups with a dentist and hygienist will indicate whether enough care is being taken of the teeth.

HYPONATRAEMIA

Concern has been raised by some sports scientists and doctors that the message to drink during a marathon has been taken to extremes. As a result, a very, very small number of marathon runners have put themselves in a potentially life-threatening position because they have developed hyponatraemia or low sodium levels in the blood. With exceptionally large intakes of water, the sodium plasma concentration in the blood falls as excessive amounts of water enter the bloodstream. Because urine production is reduced during exercise, excess water cannot be lost fast enough to bring levels back down to normal. This is compounded by sodium losses in sweat. Sodium is an essential electrolyte involved in maintaining body fluid balance and blood osmolality, and aiding muscle contractions. The faster and lower the plasma sodium concentration falls, the greater the risk to health and more serious the consequences. Ultimately, hyponatraemic encephalopathy or swelling of the brain develops, resulting in death; tragically, this happened to a female runner in the 2002 Boston Marathon. The fall in plasma sodium concentration changes the osmotic gradient across the blood–brain barrier and this leads to a rapid movement of water into the brain.

Females are at greater risk of hyponatraemia than men because they do not sweat as much, have a smaller blood volume, which is easier to overfill, and require up to 30 per cent less fluid intake than men. Most marathoners who have developed problems of hyponatraemia have been women. Runners finishing in five or more hours, particularly 'virgin' marathoners,

DEVELOPMENT OF HYPONATRAEMIA

136–142mmol sodium per litre – normal plasma sodium concentration.

125–135mmol sodium per litre – mild symptoms, including bloating, weight gain or mild nausea.

<125mmol sodium per litre – more severe symptoms, such as confusion, throbbing headache, wheezy breathing, swollen hands and feet, unusual fatigue and poor coordination.

<120mmol sodium per litre – seizure, coma and ultimately death.

AVOIDING HYPONATRAEMIA

Use a sports drink rather than water.

Avoid diluting sports drinks.

Drink early in the race and reduce intake in the later stages as pace slows up.

Let thirst dictate intake in the last miles.

Nibble on an energy bar towards the end of a marathon rather than drink water.

Determine likely sweat rate and drink enough to minimize dehydration while avoiding over-consumption.

Recognize any weight gain during training runs as a sign of excessive drinking. Reduce intake on subsequent runs.

Know warning signs and look out for them in other runners, too.

If warning signs are noticed, stop running, stop drinking and seek medical help immediately.

Include a salty snack such as Twiglets or salted pretzels as part of the refuelling process after the race and include added salt in general diet*.

Do at least three half-marathons before attempting a full marathon.

* Runners with high blood pressure who have been advised to reduce their dietary salt intake should seek advice from their doctor.

are less likely to have problems with overheating and as a result will have lower fluid requirements. However, at about 20 miles, as they tire and slow up, there is a great temptation to drink more and more in an attempt to feel better. In addition, running at this slower pace also makes it easier to manage drinks than when running at a much faster pace.

Problems of hyponatraemia are far less likely to happen on training runs, where there is less access to fluids. In some marathons, water is available every mile from very early in the race. Runners relying solely or primarily on water for fluid intake, and those who start running already mildly hyponatraemic because they have drunk excessively in the days and hours before the marathon, will be at greater risk as mild symptoms become severe. Faster runners may suffer from heat injury, especially on hot days, but not from hyponatraemia (*see* Chapter 7).

Runners need to take their fluid strategy seriously – knowing their own individual requirements in all likely running conditions, deciding early in training what will be used during the marathon, and then testing it thoroughly in training. Once a fluid plan has been devised, it should be adhered to on the day. Fluid intake should be sufficient to keep the body hydrated or at least to minimize weight loss through sweating to no more than 1 per cent of body weight. Advice is to drink enough to stay relatively hydrated but avoid excessive intakes of water.

CHAPTER 4

The Marathon Countdown

The average marathon runner needs approximately 2,800 calories to run the 26.2 miles, whatever their speed. That energy must come from the food eaten in the days leading up to the marathon and particularly from the carbohydrate content of the diet. Poor stores of muscle glycogen will limit performance and significantly affect the overall finishing time. In the non-elite runner, glycogen stores can run out after running 16 to 20 miles. When there is no longer enough stored carbohydrate to maintain running pace, runners are described as 'hitting the wall'. They slow up, start walking or even stop, feeling as if their legs are made of lead and that they have absolutely no energy left. They may even feel dizzy and confused.

PREPARATION

A runner's preparation for the race, in terms of diet, fluid intake, sleep, rest and training in the week leading up to marathon, is vital, but plans must be made well in advance and, crucially, must have been practised prior to the race. Nothing should be left to chance. Marathon organizers, particularly of the larger races, provide plenty of useful information that participants would do well to heed. For example, it can be reassuring to find out that there are plenty of lavatories at the start. However, given the number of runners, there may still be long queues and this needs to be taken in account when drawing up the marathon day plan. Similarly, it is good to know that although

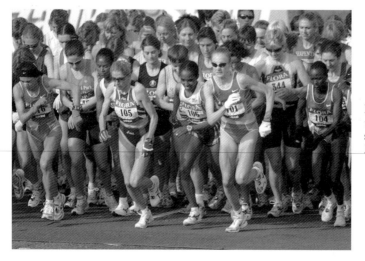

Paula Radcliffe (*front right with sunglasses*) sets off at the start of the Flora London Marathon 2003. (EMPICS)

lavatories en route may be limited, they will be well signed. Finding out the intervals between the water and sports-drink stations will be necessary to draw up a fluid strategy that will minimize dehydration, but also avoid the rare but possible risk of hyponatraemia.

Planning the Preparation

It is important never to do something for the first time on race day, so the meal the night before the race and the pre-race meal should be worked out and then practised as part of longer runs leading up to the marathon itself. Having found out what brand of sports drink is going to be available along the route, runners should use this drink during training runs. On longer runs, this may involve running a looped circuit, past home or perhaps a friend's house, where full bottles can be picked up every thirty minutes or so. Alternatively, bribing a friend or relative to cycle alongside will allow drinks to be handed over at regular intervals. A sports drink, even just a different brand or flavour, should never be used for the first time during the marathon. If a runner is not used to the drink, it could cause problems; at the very least, it could make the race a less than pleasant experience; at worst, it could lead to a withdrawal from the race. It may be necessary to use a different drink in half-marathon races but this will be less of a problem.

The pre-race meal should be eaten three to four hours before the start. For a 9.00am start, this means eating at 6.00am or even earlier. Runners need to practise this a few times by incorporating it into the training programme. This is particularly important for those who normally do the majority of their mileage in the evening. Half-marathons can be used as dress rehearsals. During 5km and 10km races there is no need for extra carbohydrate to be consumed while running, as stores will not be depleted during the race.

However, drinking a sports drink will certainly do no harm and again can be part of the rehearsal for the big day. In half-marathon events, runners can experiment with using sports drinks alone, gels with water, or a combination of both to see what suits them best. Some runners like to top up fuel supplies with 'solid' food such as energy bars, dried fruit (dates, raisins and apricots) or jelly sweets, which can easily be carried in a bum bag. Sticky items should be avoided as they can collect fluff and leave the fingers feeling uncomfortable. Others prefer to suck boiled sweets, as they release sugars slowly, but obviously care must be taken not to choke while running. Taking in carbohydrate in this form does not remove the need to take on board fluids; in fact, fluids will help the swallowing process, speed up digestion and, of course, help to minimize dehydration. An intake of 350 to 500ml of water per energy bar is suggested and runners should nibble on a bar rather than try to eat a whole bar in one go.

In the final week, runners often experience aches and pains. These may be nothing more than tight muscles, which a good massage will alleviate. Those who are carrying niggling injuries or an illness would be well advised to consider postponing the race and either running one at a later date or if possible getting an automatic entry for the following year (see Chapter 7). It is common to feel restless and full of energy as training is tapered down in the week of the race but the temptation to train, cross-train or even do physically active things such as gardening or DIY must be resisted. Large marathons, such as the London race, hold exhibitions during the days leading up to the race and this is usually where runners have to register and collect their running numbers. Walking around the exhibition for several hours, particularly the day before the race, is not advisable, as it can be very tiring. If possible, competitors should register on the first day of the exhibition. If they have to register the day before the race, they should aim to do this as early as they can. Minimum time spent at the exhibition will leave most of the day to rest and relax. The weekend should be organized to avoid or at the very least minimize any last-minute stresses.

Contents of the race-day kit bag should be checked and double-checked before being laid out the day before the race, allowing time to buy any items that are found to be missing. Some items will depend on the weather forecast – for example, bin liners and a change of clothing for a wet day, and old woolly hat, gloves and top (which can be discarded once into the race) when the forecast is for cold weather. Looser clothing that 'breathes' is better for hot days. Be prepared for all possible weather conditions so that there are no last-minute panics. Including a variety of snacks will allow the runner to choose a food that appeals after the marathon. Snacks may be provided by the race organizers

---

POSSIBLE FUEL AND FLUID ITEMS FOR THE KIT BAG

Sandwiches, filled rolls or bagels.

Fresh fruit – bananas, seedless grapes.

Dried fruit – raisins, apricots, dates.

Jaffa Cakes, fig rolls, digestive biscuits.

Simple cake, such as scones, pancakes, Swiss roll, malt loaf, iced buns, fingers, currant buns and so on.

Cereal bars.

Sports/energy bars and gels.

Boiled sweets, jelly sweets, jelly beans.

Sports drink.

Water.

---

but they are not always suitable, or familiar to every runner.

The Last Few Days

In the last days before the race it is important to have foods that are familiar. For runners staying at home or with friends this will not be a problem, but, for those in hotels or bed and breakfast accommodation, care will be needed. An enquiry at the time of booking about meals and mealtimes will help in planning what extras need to be packed before leaving home. This way, the risk of last-minute dietary problems should be minimized. Familiar food eaten in hygienic places is an important component of successful marathon preparation. Sufficient fluids should be drunk, to ensure that runners are fully hydrated by race day. Again, being away from home and the normal daily routine may lead to a reduced fluid intake. Runners should keep a check on their urinating habits – regularly passing pale, plentiful urine can be taken as a reasonable sign of hydration.

CARBOHYDRATE LOADING

The Research

Carbohydrate loading is by no means a new technique. The original research by Christensen and Hansen, which firmly established the relationship between a high-carbohydrate diet and improved endurance capacity, was reported as long ago as 1939. They looked at the exercise tolerance of a group of subjects on a cycle ergometer after they had followed different diets for three to four days – a normal mixed diet, a diet containing fat and protein, and a high-carbohydrate diet. After the high-carbohydrate diet, the endurance capacity of the subjects almost doubled compared with their performance following the normal mixed diet. The high-fat/high-protein diet, on the other hand, reduced exercise performance to almost half that of the subjects following the normal mixed diet.

Studies carried out in the early 1960s were able to make use of muscle biopsy techniques. As a result, two Swedish clinicians, Bergstrom and Hultman, were able to show that fatigue in endurance exercise (cycling in this case) was associated with the fall in muscle glycogen in the exercising muscles. Their subsequent experiments, published in 1966, were to shape the concept of carbohydrate loading. Using a specially adapted cycle ergometer, with two seats side by side, they pedalled with one leg each while resting the other. Having pedalled to exhaustion and taken muscle biopsies from each other, they found that they both had very low levels of muscle glycogen in the exercised legs. Continuing to take biopsies for three more days, they were then able to show not only that the muscle glycogen stores in the exercising legs had returned to normal resting levels after one day, but also that, after three days, muscle glycogen levels were two to three times the normal resting level. This was achieved while following a diet high in carbohydrate. Consuming a diet high in fat and protein but low in carbohydrate did not restore glycogen levels even after several days.

Further studies by other researchers showed that high levels of muscle glycogen did not affect speed at the start of exercise, but did allow pace to be maintained for longer. In other words, the point at which fatigue caused the runner to slow pace occurred later, leading to a faster overall time. Muscle glycogen levels are normally 100 to 120mmol/kg wet weight. By carbohydrate loading, these levels can be increased to 150 to 200mmol/kg wet weight.

Traditional vs. Modified Carbohydrate Loading

Traditionally, carbohydrate loading was achieved by first exercising to exhaustion seven days before the marathon, to empty the muscle glycogen stores completely. There then followed three days of a low-carbohydrate/high-fat/high-protein diet, in amounts that met energy requirements while still continuing training. Finally, a high-carbohydrate diet – with at least 70 per cent of the total energy being provided in the form of carbohydrate – was eaten for the last three or four days before the race. This would load the muscle glycogen stores to maximum. During the last three to four days, training was tapered right down to a very light volume, to preserve muscle glycogen stores.

While popular in the 1970s, doubts began to be raised as to whether it was necessary or, indeed, harmful to include the exhaustive exercise and low-carbohydrate phase. Exercising to exhaustion close to a marathon could cause premature peaking, interfere with the training programme and increase the risk of stress injury. A low-carbohydrate diet is unpleasant and can cause irritability and lightheadedness, making training very difficult. A low-carbohydrate diet is associated with an increased risk of infection as hard training with low glycogen stores leads to an increase in stress hormones and a negative effect on the immune system. All these factors could seriously undermine confidence during preparation for a marathon.

On returning to a high-carbohydrate diet, runners often experienced gastrointestinal upsets and weight gain. It was also very easy to get the loading wrong using the traditional method, by depleting effectively but not eating enough to increase the muscle glycogen level above normal – all the unpleasantness without any gain.

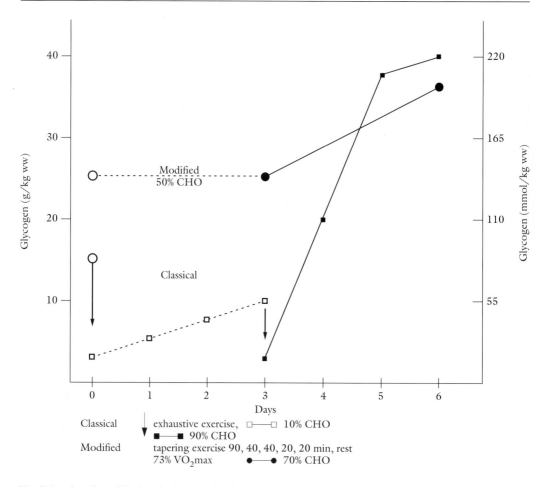

Traditional and modified carbohydrate loading.

Modified carbohydrate loading requires a gradual taper of training in the last week before the marathon, particularly in the last three days, with complete rest the day before the race. In other words, the initial depletion phase is completely omitted. At the same time, the carbohydrate content of the diet needs to be increased from five days before the race (three days may not be enough for everyone) to provide 8–10g carbohydrate per kg body weight per day. A 70kg male would therefore need 560 to 700g carbohydrate and a 55kg female, 440 to 550g carbohydrate. This can be easily worked out using 50g carbohydrate portions from carbohydrate-rich foods (*see* Chapter 2).

The emphasis must be on every meal containing a good serving of carbohydrate, with carbohydrate-rich snacks in between. Runners should avoid over-eating or stuffing themselves. At no time should they feel bloated or uncomfortable from eating. Many runners find it more practical to eat little and often. Cutting back on dietary fibre intake and making more use of concentrated sugary sources of carbohydrate can make loading a more 'comfortable' experience. Eating a high-carbohydrate diet is not an excuse to eat large amounts of fat, which would lead to excessive energy intake and feelings of heaviness. A regular fluid intake is vital as glycogen is stored in the muscles in conjunction with water (1g glycogen being stored with 3g water).

Loading with carbohydrate means there will be an overall increase in body weight of approximately 2kg so runners who are sensitive about their weight should avoid the bathroom scales. In the early stages of the race, a runner may feel heavy, but this soon wears off and any negative aspects are far outweighed by the benefits of starting the race with full stores of muscle glycogen and a well-hydrated body. Certainly, by the end of the marathon, the extra weight (and maybe even more) will have gone.

Modified carbohydrate loading is particularly valuable for the first-time marathon runner and non-elite runner, who are both at greater risk of running out of carbohydrate stores than the highly trained experienced elite runner. Even so, carbohydrate loading appears to work only for a well-trained runner. Loading after a training programme that has provided inadequate preparation for a marathon (for example, low weekly mileage and no half-marathon races) will not make any significant difference to endurance capacity. Consuming extra carbohydrate will not increase muscle glycogen stores unless the enzymes in the muscles have been primed by a good training programme. Sadly, with inadequate preparation, extra carbohydrate will simply be stored as fat.

More recently, it has been shown that carbohydrate loading for just one day may be enough to ensure full stores of muscle glycogen in well-trained runners. Researchers have shown that runners who consumed 10.2g carbohydrate per kg body weight in the twenty-four hours prior to the marathon, while remaining totally inactive, significantly boosted their carbohydrate stores. This may be of value for that very small minority who have to train right up to the day before the marathon. However, for the vast majority, the modified loading with gradual training taper allows the body to recover from the training load, while ensuring that carbohydrate stores are maximized. It is certainly worth trying out a carbohydrate-loading regime in one or two of the longer runs – runs over 25km (15 miles) – prior to the marathon itself.

It is also worth noting that carbohydrate loading prior to exercise is considerably less effective in raising muscle glycogen stores in females than in males, and is also affected by the stage in the menstrual cycle (*see* Chapter 6). Female runners should still follow the moderate loading advice but they must also be aware of the increased importance of taking on board carbohydrate in drinks during the marathon. They should, of course, have previously used such drinks during long training runs and half-marathon races.

THE DAY BEFORE THE RACE

Eating

All foods eaten on this day should be foods normally included in the daily diet. This is not the time to start experimenting with anything new. Attention should be paid to optimizing fluid and salt levels in the body by keeping up a good/regular intake of fluid and adding salt to food. This is especially important in warm/hot conditions.

Most foods eaten traditionally at breakfast time are suitable, although a full English fried breakfast is certainly not a wise choice. It is carbohydrate not protein (and definitely not fat) that is important at this time. Cereals with low-fat milk, bread, toast, rolls, bagels, crumpets with low-fat spread, jam, marmalade or honey, fruit and yoghurt and plenty of fluids, including fruit juice, are all suitable. Lunch can be built around sandwiches with a variety of breads and low-fat fillings, jacket potatoes with tuna (in brine or spring water), cottage cheese or baked beans (if wind is not a problem), or pasta or rice salads (no oily dressings), finishing with fruit, yoghurt and more fluids. The last meal of the day should be a familiar one based around pasta, rice or potatoes, with a small amount of chicken, tuna, very lean red meat or a low-fat vegetarian alternative. Meat should not be high on the menu and hotdogs, hamburgers and kebabs should certainly be avoided, especially ones bought from mobile catering establishments. An upset stomach causes dehydration, which can become a serious health risk during the marathon. Vegetables can be included, but at this stage are not essential. Many runners just prefer to have a tomato-based sauce with pasta or rice for this meal.

Portions need not be large but the emphasis should be very much on the carbohydrate content of the meal. This is particularly important for those who are already feeling nervous and know they will not be able to face food on the morning of the race. Those who do need to eat more in the evening can top up with fruit, low-fat rice pudding, yoghurts and bread. Indeed, anything high in carbohydrate but low in fat that is tempting and familiar will be fine. Curries and spicy dishes generally, together with high-fibre foods, seafood, fatty foods, rare meat and gas-producing foods such as beans should be avoided. Many runners have regretted their choice of meal the night before once the digestive system wakes up in the morning and the pre-race nerves start.

The evening meal should not be eaten too late. If hunger pangs do kick in later, toast and jam, hot milk with biscuits, or a small bowl of cereal and milk should fill the gap without causing any problems. Ideally, the day should be fairly restful and most runners will find that they do not need to have snacks between meals. Fluid intake should be maintained throughout the evening.

Sleeping

Mild sleep deprivation or one night of almost total sleeplessness before a race seems to have little effect on physical performance, but those who are worried that nerves may disrupt sleep patterns the night before the marathon should try to get a few early nights in the week leading up to the race. That way, they should be less concerned if they do not sleep well the night before. Making the last meal before bed a high-carbohydrate meal (which it should be) helps to increase the body's production of the hormone serotonin, which induces sleep. There is also some truth in the old wives' tale that a milky drink sweetened with honey encourages sleep, again because of the effect of the carbohydrate on serotonin production. Having camomile tea at bedtime instead of coffee or tea, and sprinkling a little oil of lavender on the pillow may also have a soporific effect. Creating the right environment for sleep by making it quiet (this may mean using earplugs), dark, cool and comfortable (a good mattress and pillow help) may make the night more restful.

Alcohol has diuretic properties and in most situations the recommendation would be to avoid it at this stage. In practice, some runners find that a small drink is relaxing, particularly when sleeping in unfamiliar surroundings. In this case, having a pint (half for females) of ordinary beer or lager (no strong varieties), but no more, will not be a problem, but spirits and wine should be avoided. Having a non-alcoholic drink afterwards will counter any dehydrating effects of the alcohol.

EATING AND DRINKING ON RACE DAY

Pre-Race Meal

A good diet in the previous days will have already ensured the muscle glycogen stores are full. This meal provides an opportunity to top up the liver glycogen stores which will have been used or partially used up during the night and to replace the energy used since the last meal (probably between 400–600kcal). The meal will also help to prevent hunger pangs and leave the stomach feeling settled and comfortable. However, the meal must be kept low in fat, otherwise food will remain in the stomach too long and lead to subsequent discomfort. At this stage, there is no need to worry too much about other nutrients such as vitamins and minerals. Fluids and, to a lesser extent, food will help to rehydrate the body. Knowing that the planned dietary and fluid preparation have been completed can help psychologically, making the runner feel alert and ready for the start of the race.

The exact choice of food will depend on what is available and what the runner finds comfortable, familiar and enjoyable. Nutritionally, the meal should be rich in carbohydrates, ideally with a low glycaemic index, low in fat, low or moderate in protein and low in fibre. Such a balance of nutrients will ensure that the food has left the stomach (fat and protein take longer to leave the stomach than carbohydrate) and has been digested before the start of the race. Those runners who cannot face food may be able to tolerate a liquid meal, an energy bar and a drink, or just an energy drink. Most marathons start in the morning and runners eating away from home should find out what foods will be available when they need them, possibly as early as 5.00am. Not all types of accommodation will be geared up to provide a meal at this time, particularly on a Sunday, which is a popular day for

SUITABLE PRE-MARATHON FOODS
Breakfast cereals, including porridge with low-fat milk, sliced banana or dried fruit.
Toast with low-fat spread, jam, honey or marmalade.
Pancakes with syrup.
Toasted muffins (English not American!), crumpets or pikelets, with honey and sliced banana.
Banana and honey sandwiches.
Low-fat rice pudding.
Low-fat yoghurt.
Canned spaghetti in tomato sauce on toast.

marathon races. Runners may need to take their own emergency rations, including any dishes or utensils that are needed. Fortunately, most foods that are suitable for this meal tend to travel well and do not present any major storage or preparation problems.

The actual time that breakfast needs to be eaten depends on travel time to the start, what time the race starts and the time needed to get organized at the start (deposit kit bag, go to the loo, stretch and so on). This should have been worked out well in advance so that the whole process can be tried out at least once before the day itself. The last meal should ideally be eaten at least three hours before the start.

Before the Start

Depending on the length of time from leaving home to the start of the race, some runners may need a snack en route, such as a sandwich or cereal bar. However, care should be taken not to over-eat. It has been suggested that an intake of 1–2g carbohydrate per kg body weight should be consumed one hour before the start, either as a low-GI food or a drink made up primarily of glucose polymers, followed by 180ml of sports drink ten minutes before the start. This regime should maintain a good flow of fluid and carbohydrate from the stomach to the muscles.

Others suggest taking regular sips of a sports drink from two hours before the race starts until thirty minutes before the start – this should allow time to urinate out any excess. Precise timing will be required for this, particularly at a marathon with a large number of entrants, where there may be long queues for the lavatories.

Just five minutes before the start a final top-up of approx 50ml of sports drink will provide reassurance that both fluid and fuel reserves are as full as is practically possible, without leading to worries that early into the race there will be a need to find a lavatory.

During the Marathon

The role of fluid intake during a marathon has gained in importance over the years, and the International Association of Athletics Federation (IAAF) guidelines on fluid intake during long-distance running have changed accordingly:

- 1953: water every 5km after 15km;
- 1967: water every 5km after 11km;
- 1977: water every 2.4km after 5km;
- 1990: water and/or carbohydrate drink every 3km.

As many runners will run out of stores of muscle glycogen before the end of the marathon, choosing a sports drink that contains 6 to 7 per cent carbohydrate (such as Lucozade Sport, Gatorade or Powerade), or using carbohydrate gels plus water, will not only help to minimize dehydration but will also top up ever-depleting carbohydrate stores. Some runners try to avoid eating and drinking during the race in the hope that they will not need to make a pit-stop. This is a false time economy, as running pace will inevitably get progressively slower. Other runners wait until they feel thirsty or tired before they start taking on board fluids. Taking regular amounts of sports drinks at each drinking station can help to avoid the unpleasant effects

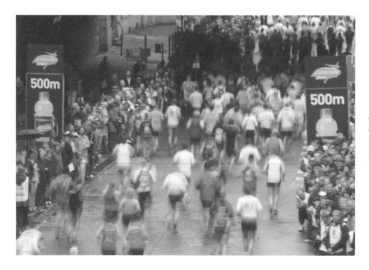

Alert for the next Lucozade Sport station at the Flora London Marathon 2004.
(GETTY IMAGES)

WATER-STATION ETIQUETTE

Go for the less crowded areas – usually at the end of the water station rather than at the beginning.

Go to stations on the left as they should also be less crowded – right-handed runners tend to go to the right and, of course, there are more right-handed than left-handed people.

Get away from the station before starting to drink – there will be less chance of being jostled.

If drinks are provided in cups, pinch the sides together as this will be easier to drink and more comfortable to hold.

Reduce running speed when drinking, even to a walking pace – it reduces the risk of choking or the drink going up the nose. The extra time is hardly going to affect finishing time.

Take care when throwing away empty cups, bottles or sports packs.

A Lucozade Sport station at the Flora London Marathon 2004. (GETTY IMAGES)

of 'hitting the wall'. Waiting until the latter stages of the race is not advisable; the 'wall' will be 'hit' and performance will suffer. Drinking early on in the race may also help in preventing cramps later in the race; these are particularly common in runners who have not trained enough or who have become dehydrated.

The International Marathon Medical Directors Association (IMMDA) was formed in 1984 to promote and study the health of long-distance runners; to promote research into the cause and treatment of running injuries; to prevent the occurrence of injuries during mass-participation runs; to offer guidelines for the provision of uniform marathon medical services throughout the world; and to promote a close working relationship between race and medical directors in achieving these four goals. In November 2001, the IMMDA Advisory Statement on Guidelines for fluid replacement during marathon running was unanimously approved at the IMMDA General Assembly. One of the guidelines in the statement was 'Runners should aim to drink ad libitum between 400–800ml per hour, with the higher rates for the faster, heavier runners competing in warm environmental conditions and the lower rates for the slower runners/walkers completing marathon races in cooler environmental conditions.' The full statement can be found at their website:

www.aims-association.org/immda.htm

The best-known advice on exercise and fluid replacement comes, however, from the American College of Sports Medicine (ACMS) in their Position Stand published in 1996. Their advice seems somewhat at variance with the IMMDA advice:

1. It is recommended that individuals consume a nutritionally balanced diet and drink adequate fluids during the 24-hour period before an event, especially during the period that includes the meal prior to exercise, to promote proper hydration before exercise or competition.

2. It is recommended that individuals drink about 500ml of fluid about 2 hours before exercise to promote adequate hydration and allow time for excretion of excess ingested water.

3. During exercise, athletes should start drinking early and at regular intervals in an attempt to consume fluids at a rate sufficient to replace all the water lost through sweating (i.e. body weight loss), or consume the maximal amount that can be tolerated.

4. It is recommended that ingested fluids be cooler than ambient temperature and flavoured to enhance palatability and promote fluid replacement. Fluids should be readily available and served in containers that allow adequate volumes to be ingested with ease and with minimal interruption of exercise.

5. Addition of proper amounts of carbohydrates and/or electrolytes to a fluid replacement solution is recommended for exercise events of duration greater than 1 h since it does not significantly impair water delivery to the body and may enhance performance. During exercise lasting less than 1 h, there is little evidence of physiological or physical performance differences between consuming a carbohydrate-electrolyte drink and plain water.

6. During intense exercise lasting longer than 1 h, it is recommended that carbohydrates are ingested at a rate of 30–60g per h to maintain oxidation of carbohydrates and delay fatigue. This rate of carbohydrate intake can be achieved without compromising fluid delivery by drinking 600–1200ml per h of solutions containing 4–8 per cent carbohydrates (4–8g per 100ml). The carbohydrates can be sugars (glucose or sucrose) or starch (e.g. maltodextrin).

7. Inclusion of sodium (0.5-0.7g per litre of water) in the rehydration solution ingested during exercise lasting longer than 1 h is recommended since it may be advantageous in enhancing palatability, promoting fluid retention, and possibly preventing hyponatraemia in certain individuals who drink excessive quantities of fluid.

(REFERENCE: American College of Sports Medicine. Position Stand: Exercise and fluid replacement. *Medicine and Science in Sports and Exercise* vol. 28, no. i–vii, 1996.)

It should now be clear to runners, particularly those preparing to run their first marathon, that it is vital to experiment in training with different fluids and quantities, to find out which fluid strategy suits them best. This strategy can then be rehearsed over and over again in all training runs over an hour. What works best in training is what should be used in the marathon itself.

Runners need to work out their own fluid requirements based on their training runs and estimated fluid losses but general advice is to drink little and often (*see* Chapter 3). Thirst is not a good indicator of hydration status so, rather than waiting to feel thirsty, runners should consume fluids regularly and increase the intake if the weather is hot. Even on cool days, marathon runners can lose a lot of fluid through sweating.

Runners should aim to take in 30–60g of carbohydrate per hour. As most isotonic sports drinks contain 6 to 7 per cent carbohydrate, an approximate intake of 500ml or 1,000ml per

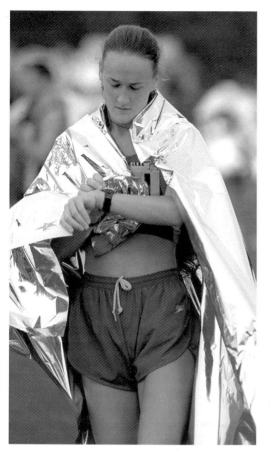

A competitor checks her finishing time. (EMPICS)

hour will provide 30 or 60g of carbohydrate per hour respectively. Runners using gels (carried in a bum bag) should open the pack and start swallowing just before a water station, then pick up some water and aim to drink 250–350ml per gel pack, to wash down the gel and rehydrate.

After the Marathon

By the end of the marathon, runners will have almost, or totally, depleted their stores of muscle glycogen, they will probably be dehydrated to varying degrees, and will certainly have

sore muscles. It is important to keep walking once the finishing line has been crossed. This will keep the blood pumping around the legs and help to stop painful cramps and sore legs over the following days. Standing around at the finish, runners can soon get cold as heat will continue to be lost from the body. A tracksuit or sweater should be put on as soon as possible. This is when the bag-carrying friends or family come into their own; they can also offer the snacks and drinks that should have been packed in the kit bag the day before.

Runners should aim to consume 200–300kcal in the first twenty minutes after finishing and then enjoy small, regular intakes of food throughout the rest of the day. Sandwiches with a protein filling will provide approximately 70 per cent of the calories as carbohydrate and 30 per cent as protein, which is a pretty good ratio. One of the best choices of sandwich filling is salmon (smoked or otherwise) and salad, as the fish contains omega-3 fatty acids and antioxidants, nutrients that can help to minimize post-race damage and soreness.

Fluid intake should be maintained after the race is over and, indeed, throughout the rest of the day. Sports drinks (which are usually handed out at the finish) continue to be a good choice, as they hydrate and refuel at the same time. They should be used until urinating habits return to normal. Feeling too tired to eat and drink is no excuse; food and fluids are the two main things that will perk up an exhausted runner.

Many runners will want to celebrate with an alcoholic drink. Ideally, this should be postponed until full rehydration has been achieved. For those who cannot wait, an ordinary beer or lager (with perhaps a lemonade top?) is a much better choice than wine or spirits. Matching an alcoholic drink with a sports drink, soft drink or water will help to keep the rehydration process going. Many

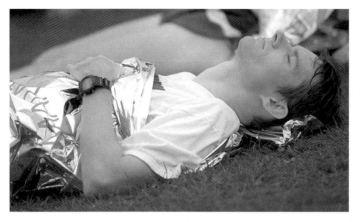

A competitor enjoys a well-deserved lie-down after completing the course. (EMPICS)

POST-MARATHON MEAL CHOICES

Pizza – vegetarian or margherita with no extra cheese.

Indian – plain rice with tandoori chicken dish or a mild vegetable curry.

Chinese – plain rice with chicken in lemon sauce or bean curd stir-fry.

Italian – spaghetti napoletana.

Greek – plain rice with lamb, pepper and onion kebab, or vegetarian stuffed peppers or tomatoes.

Pub – jacket potato with baked beans or shepherd's pie.

---

only the marathon itself but also of all the training leading up to the big day. A couple of light runs will do no harm but the emphasis must be on relaxing, with plenty of stretching and no rigorous exercise. It is important to keep away from people with infections. Marathon runners are six times more likely to pick up an infection in the week after running a marathon, because the immune system will be suppressed. Staying relaxed, maintaining a diet high in antioxidants, sleeping well and practising good hygiene will all help to keep infections at bay.

Maintaining a diet high in carbohydrate and protein will help the recovery process but it is important to remember that the body will not need the same amount of energy (food), so portions and snacking should be trimmed back. Runners will have struck the pavement an average of fifty to seventy times a minute with each foot during the marathon. From start to finish, this translates into the feet making contact with the ground some 50,000 times. This continuous hammering breaks down red blood cells in the blood in the feet and reduces the overall level of haemoglobin in the blood. In the days and weeks after the marathon, it is therefore important to maintain a good intake of dietary iron (*see* Chapter 2).

runners will be eating on their way home and even at this stage it will pay off in the days to come to make wise choices.

THE DAYS FOLLOWING RACE DAY

It is important to have plenty of rest and sleep in the days after running a marathon, to allow the body to recover from the stresses of not

TRAVELLING

Eating and Drinking

Runners may have to travel a couple of hours by car, take a six-hour train or coach journey, or even fly for several hours across time zones to compete in a marathon. It is essential that, whatever the mode of transport or travel time, planning and preparation take into account what will be eaten and drunk while in transit. Travelling by car, train or bus should not present too many problems, particularly if the assumption is made that it is better to take food and fluids rather than rely on what might be available en route. Food and fluids for the journey simply need to be added into the overall preparation for the marathon. As refuelling after the marathon takes not just hours but days, planning and preparation must also include the post-marathon diet while travelling home, too.

SUITABLE FOODS AND FLUIDS FOR TRAVELLING

Fresh fruit	Water
Dried fruit	Fruit juice
Dried fruit and nuts	Ready to drink squash
Cereal and breakfast bars	Sports drinks
Sports/energy bars	

Breakfast cereal (eaten by the handful)

Sandwiches, rolls, bagels

Breadsticks, pretzels, crackers

Fig rolls, ginger biscuits (particularly useful for alleviating travel sickness)

Malt loaf, pancakes, scones, Chelsea buns, etc.

Long hours of travelling, by any method, can upset the digestive system, particularly leading to constipation. Runners who recognize this as a potential problem should make sure they eat plenty of fruit, include some fibre-rich foods, and drink plenty of water, but care will be needed not to overdo things. Taking this advice to the extreme may well cause the opposite effect during the race itself. When travelling, it is all too easy to either under-eat (not feeling hungry) or over-eat (less active, bored), so attention needs to be paid to quantity as well as quality of food consumed. Jotting down what is eaten and drunk, and when, can help in keeping to the marathon diet plan. Runners should try to get up, move around and stretch if possible during the journey, particularly as it only takes two hours before the body starts getting stiff, blood begins to pool in the legs and travel fatigue kicks in.

Air Travel

Hydration and Food

Air in an aircraft cabin is very dry (low humidity) and this increases the risk of dehydration. A lip salve can help prevent lips becoming dry and sore and those who normally wear contact lenses may find it more comfortable to wear glasses during a flight. Dehydration can be avoided or minimized by increasing fluid intake, avoiding alcohol completely from the start of the journey, and drinking no more than the usual intake of caffeine-containing drinks such as tea, coffee and some soft drinks (particularly colas and energy drinks). More emphasis should be placed on drinking bottled water, juices and caffeine-free soft drinks. Still rather than sparkling mineral water is probably a better choice as the bubbles have to go somewhere and could cause discomfort. At least a litre of water carried in hand luggage can help to maintain fluid intake between landing and reaching your destination.

With sufficient notice, special meals, such as vegetarian, Kosher or wheat-free, can be ordered. The range of meals does vary between airlines. Meal portions tend to be on the small side, certainly in economy class, so it may be necessary to bulk this up with supplies from home carried on board in hand luggage. Extra fruit is always a good idea as this will help to keep the bowels working; air travel does tend to encourage sluggishness in this area. Any left-over fruit may have to be dumped before customs as many countries do not allow importation of fresh fruit. Indeed, it is worth checking out all regulations before travelling, as there may be restrictions on other food items.

DVT and Jet Lag

Sitting on a plane in a cramped, confined space can cause stiffness and muscle cramps. Runners should heed the warnings about developing deep vein thrombosis (DVT) and take all necessary precautions in-flight.

Sleep should be attempted if it will be night-time at the final destination, or if life has been hectic in the days leading up to departure and the runner is suffering from sleep deprivation. Sleeping during the flight when it is daytime at the destination could make further sleep difficult on arrival. Ways to keep awake include talking to other travellers (provided they are happy to listen), watching in-flight movies or playing video games. If it is night-time on arrival, it is sensible to get to bed as quickly as possible. On the other hand, if it is daytime, sleep should be limited to an hour's nap followed by a quick, cool shower. This should help to wake up a weary traveller.

The body clock promotes activity in the daytime and uninterrupted sleep at night. In normal circumstances, the body clock remains stable and is not adjusted by transient changes in the environment or lifestyle of the individual. However, crossing a number of time zones plays havoc with the body clock resulting in the well-known symptoms of jet lag. A runner may feel tired in the daytime at the destination and still find it difficult to sleep at night-time. It becomes much harder to concentrate on anything and people suffering from jet lag tend to find it very hard to motivate themselves. Research has shown that mental and physical performance are definitely decreased as a result of jet lag.

Other symptoms of jet lag include an increase in incidence of headaches, loss of appetite, changes in bowel movements and an overall feeling of general irritability. In general, the symptoms get worse as more time zones are crossed, but some individuals appear to cope better than others. Younger runners tend to be more flexible in their habits and will probably adjust better than older runners. Those who enjoy getting up in the morning will find it easier to adjust to an eastward shift than

---

MINIMIZING THE RISK OF DVT, STIFFNESS AND CRAMPING IN-FLIGHT

Book a seat near the exit or aisle to give more space to move legs around.

Avoid sitting with crossed legs or obstructions around the calves, otherwise blood flow can be restricted.

Wear loose-fitting baggy clothes to avoid restricting circulation.

Take shoes off for the duration of the flight.

Wear support or compression stockings.

Walk, stretch and do the exercises suggested in the in-flight magazines.

Keep up fluid intake.

---

those who prefer to stay up late. The opposite will apply to a journey in the other direction. People who find it relatively easy to get to sleep and are not affected by sleeping conditions, such as a strange bed, noisy atmosphere or other people snoring, will also be less affected. However, those who find it hard to ignore tiredness, and have difficulty in keeping going once fatigue sets in, will suffer more. People who are physically fit tend to have less difficulty adjusting than unfit travellers. This is obviously good news for runners.

If a runner plans to stay just a few days, literally flying in, running the marathon and flying home again, there will be insufficient time for the body clock to adjust. The normal practice, as adopted by airline staff, is to try as much as possible to stay in the home time zone. Flying east, this would mean that afternoon/evening would coincide with daytime at home and the morning with evening at home. A marathon run in the morning would therefore be equivalent to running at nighttime. Flying west, activities would be best carried out in the morning. A longer stay in the time zone before the race will allow adjustment of the body clock to local time.

Melatonin ingestion and avoiding exposure to bright light are both ways of minimizing the effects of jet lag. For more information, runners are referred to *Journal of Sports Sciences*, 2003, 22, 946–966, for an excellent article entitled 'The stress of travel' by Waterhouse, Reilly and Edwards.

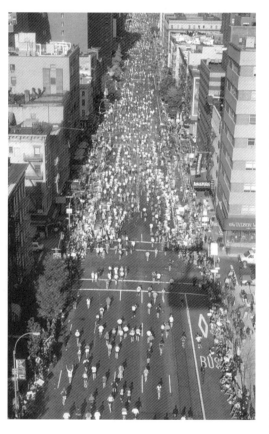

New York City Marathon 2001. (EMPICS)

ADJUSTING TO LOCAL TIME

Start to live in the destination time or stopover time as soon as the plane has taken off, by changing watch time immediately on boarding.

Adjust to the meal, bedtime and waking time at the destination immediately and resist the temptation to think about the time back home.

Use the window in the day when waking time at home overlaps with the destination waking time to do any light training.

Big heavy meals should be avoided late at night as they may make sleep even more difficult. Intake of caffeine-containing drinks should be no more than normal.

Although alcohol may help to induce sleep, it does have diuretic properties. Needing to get up in the night to pass urine might make getting back to sleep difficult.

Avoiding Stomach Upsets Abroad

Staying in a foreign country brings with it the risk of an upset stomach if attention is not paid to food safety and personal hygiene. Stomach upsets lead to dehydration and runners unlucky enough to go down with a serious bout of gastroenteritis, and who become severely dehydrated as a result, will certainly not be able to take part in the marathon. There are several things that a runner can do to minimize the risk of an upset stomach. If the local water is not safe to drink, then bottled, boiled or sterilized water must be used – always checking to make sure that the seal on the bottle has not been broken. This water should be used even for cleaning teeth. Even if the tap water is safe, travellers often still use bottled water, as the variation in the water can cause a gastrointestinal upset. Care must be taken not to ingest unsafe water in other ways so advice is not to use ice cubes and to avoid swallowing water when showering or swimming. Fruits that need peeling such as bananas and citrus fruit will be safer, and salads should only be eaten if they have been washed in clean water. Unpasteurized milk, cream, yoghurt and ice-cream should be avoided.

Well-cooked foods are safer than raw or undercooked foods and, if there is any suspicion of food having been inadequately reheated, this should be avoided. If meals are to be eaten away from the accommodation, recommendations should be sought from the hotel manager or people who know the area very well. Food sold on the street, from stalls or in open markets, should be avoided. The utmost care should be taken if shellfish is on the menu; in a Mediterranean country or a tropical climate, it may have been harvested in water that is contaminated.

Running a marathon abroad may present problems which make the dietary preparations less than perfect. Non-perishable items brought from home, such as breakfast cereal and dried milk, cereal/sport/energy bars, rice cakes and spreads, and dried fruit and nuts, can be used to supplement meals. However, it is important to check there are no import restrictions on any of these items.

CHAPTER 5
Ergogenic Supplements

Sportsmen and women use supplements for a variety of reasons: to maintain health, promote tissue growth and repair, boost immune function, gain muscle or burn fat, improve recovery, improve performance, gain advantage, because everyone else does, as a form of health insurance, because the advertisements sound convincing, or because they have been advised to do so by a friend, family member or member of their coaching or support team. Nutritional supplements include carbohydrate powders, gels and bars, protein powders and shakes, meal replacements, fluid-replacement drinks, and vitamin and mineral supplements. They are usually used because they are convenient, providing a measured dosage of a specific nutrient or nutrients. Some are used to promote general health. A runner might choose to take a one-a-day multivitamin and mineral supplement as an insurance policy in case the diet is not always providing the full range of these nutrients in sufficient amounts. Alternatively, a sports drink might be used as a convenient and easy way of keeping hydrated, or an energy bar used to refuel immediately after a training run. For more on this, *see* previous chapters.

Ergogenic supplements are used to enhance performance rather than health. They are used in the belief (correct in some cases, but not in others) that they may raise performance above expectations. This chapter covers only a selection of legal ergogenic supplements for endurance athletes.

RULES AND REGULATIONS

In May 2003, a position statement was published on behalf of UK Sport, the British Olympic Association (BOA), the British Paralympic Association (BPA), National Sports Medicine Institute (NSMI) and the Home Country Sports Councils (HCSC). The following is an extract from the statement; the statement can be viewed in full at www.uksport.gov.uk

Advice to UK Athletes on the Use of Supplements
UK athletes are strongly advised to be extremely cautious about the use of any supplements. No guarantee can be given that any particular supplement, including vitamins and minerals, ergogenic aids, and herbal remedies, is free from prohibited substances, as these products are not licensed and are not subject to the same strict manufacturing and labelling requirements as licensed medicines.

Anti-doping rules are based on the principle of strict liability and therefore, supplements are taken at an athlete's risk and personal responsibility.

Although the statement was aimed at the elite competing athlete, who is liable to be drug-tested on several occasions in a sporting career, its ethos is equally relevant to anybody taking part in sport.

The World Conference on Doping in Sport, held in February 1999, led to the publication of the Lausanne Declaration on Doping in Sport, which provided for the creation of an independent international anti-doping agency. In November 1999, the World Anti-Doping Agency (WADA) was established to promote and coordinate the fight against doping in sport internationally. In March 2003, WADA produced the World Anti-Doping Code. The basic rationale for this Code is that doping is fundamentally contrary to the spirit of sport, whose ethos is described in the following terms:

- ethics, fair play and honesty;
- health;
- excellence in performance;
- character and education;
- fun and joy;
- teamwork;
- dedication and commitment;
- respect for rules and laws;
- respect for self and other participants;
- courage;
- community and solidarity.

WADA has created a single list of prohibited substances and methods, revised annually. Substances and methods meeting two out of three criteria – performance enhancement, health risk, or violation of the 'spirit of sport' – will be placed on the list. Exemptions will be granted for therapeutic reasons, when a banned substance is needed in the treatment of a condition such as asthma, for example.

The first list came into effect on 1 January 2004 and made an immediate impact by removing caffeine and pseudo-ephedrine from the original International Olympic Committee (IOC) list of banned substances. The aim was to ensure that sportsmen and women who take over-the-counter cold cures, or drink cola or coffee, cannot be banned through inadvertent

use of substances that are both classified as mild stimulants. Both substances have a minor effect unless used in enormous quantities – in which case, the abuse would be apparent.

More information about WADA and the prohibited list can be found on their website (www.wada-ama.org).

EVALUATING ERGOGENIC SUPPLEMENTS

Before using any product, runners need to know if the product works and is suitable for training and competing in a marathon; if it is legal (not on the WADA Prohibited List); and if it is safe. In December 2000, The American Dietetic Association, Dietitians of Canada and the American College of Sports Medicine published a Joint Position Statement on 'Nutrition and Athletic Performance', which included guidelines for evaluating the claims of ergogenic aids:

Evaluate the scientific validity of an ergogenic claim:

Does the amount and the form of the active ingredient claimed to be present in the supplement match that used in the scientific studies on this ergogenic aid?

Does the claim made by the manufacturer of the product match the science of nutrition and exercise as you know it?

Does the ergogenic claim make sense for the sport for which the claim is made?

Evaluate the quality of the supportive evidence for using the ergogenic aid:

What evidence is given for using the ergogenic aid (testimonial vs scientific study)?

What is the quality of the science? What is the reputation of the author and the journal in which the research is published? Was the research sponsored by the manufacturer?

Does the experimental design meet the following criteria?

- hypothesis driven;
- double-blind placebo controlled;
- adequate and appropriate controls used; and
- appropriate dose of the ergogenic substance/placebo used.

What research methods were used and do they answer the questions asked? Are the methods clearly presented so the study results could be reproduced?

Are the methods clearly presented in an unbiased manner with appropriate statistical procedures, limitations addressed, and adverse events noted? Are the results physiologically feasible and do the conclusions follow from the data?

Evaluate the safety and legality of the ergogenic aid:

Is the product safe? Will its use compromise the health of a person? Does the product contain toxic or unknown substances or substances that alter nutrient metabolism? Is the substance contraindicated in people with a particular health problem?

Will use of the product preclude other important elements in performance? For example, does the product claim to replace food or good training practices?

Is the product illegal or banned by any athletic organizations?

(Position of the American Dietetic Association, Dietitians of Canada and the American College of Sport's Medicine: Nutrition and Athletic Performance. *J Am Diet Assoc.* 2000; 100: 1543–1556. With acknowledgement to the American Dietetic Association for permission to reproduce this section of the position statement.)

ERGOGENICS FOR MARATHON RUNNERS

Unlike the elite runner, who will be constantly looking for the competitive but hopefully legal edge, the vast majority of runners will only become aware of particular ergogenic supplements once their usage is widespread. The following is a brief review of a selection of ergogenic supplements that are assessed on the science behind them, on their effectiveness and on whether they are legal and safe.

Runners will be anxious to avoid banned substances and need to know that products are safe to take. There have been a number of positive drug tests in recent years that have arisen from athletes unknowingly taking a banned substance. Research from IOC-accredited laboratories has found products sold to athletes that have contained prohibited substances, although there was no indication of their presence on the label. Either there was inadvertent contamination in the manufacturing or distribution process, or the presence of the banned substance was due to a 'deliberate and criminal act'. In other words, the substance was added by the manufacturer, but not declared on the label. Results to date from two IOC laboratories have shown the presence of prohibited steroids in between 15 and 20 per cent of products tested.

BRANCHED-CHAIN AMINO ACIDS (BCAA)

These are the essential amino acids leucine, isoleucine and valine, which occur naturally in protein-rich foods. It has been suggested that BCAA may help runners to overcome central or mental fatigue. Tryptophan, another amino acid, is the precursor of serotonin, a brain transmitter that appears to depress the central nervous system, leading to symptoms of fatigue and sleepiness. As muscle glycogen levels fall during a long run, BCAA are used as a top-up energy source. Normally, BCAA block the entry of tryptophan into the brain, thus limiting serotonin formation. However, as BCAA get used up, to boost flagging energy supplies, circulating levels of these amino acids fall and as a result tryptophan is able to enter the brain and form serotonin. Theoretically, BCAA supplementation should help prevent the formation of fatigue-inducing serotonin. In fact, studies to date are equivocal.

BCAA are safe and legal (provided they are not contaminated), but high doses have caused gastrointestinal problems such as pain and diarrhoea. Consuming sufficient carbohydrate and good-quality protein in the daily diet, and using a sports drinks containing carbohydrate during long training runs, half-marathons and the marathon itself, are tried, tested and enjoyable ways of preventing or at least delaying the onset of fatigue.

Caffeine

Caffeine and related methylxanthine compounds are found in tea, coffee, cocoa, colas and other soft drinks, chocolate, energy drinks and some over-the-counter medicines (cold and flu remedies, pain relief products, antihistamine tablets and diuretics). Although common in the diet, caffeine is not a nutrient but a pharmacological agent.

Caffeine appears to have many actions that might enhance endurance performance. It has a direct effect on the central nervous system, influencing psychological state, particularly perception of effort and fatigue. It stimulates free fatty acid mobilization and spares the body's limited muscle glycogen stores, thus helping to delay fatigue during prolonged exercise such as distance running. It also helps in the release of calcium from muscle cells, thereby stimulating muscle contractions more effectively.

CAFFEINE CONTENT OF BEVERAGES AND FOODS (MAFF, 1998)

Product	Portion size	Caffeine (mg per serving)
Tea (loose tea)	150ml cup	10–55
	250ml mug	16–91
Tea (tea bags)	150ml cup	24–42
	250ml mug	40–70
Coffee (instant)	150ml cup	31–85
	250ml mug	52–85
Coffee (filtered/percolated)	150ml cup	46–94
	250ml mug	76–157
Coffee (decaffeinated)	150ml cup	<2
Cola	330ml can	11–70
	500ml bottle	16–106
Stimulant drinks	250ml bottle	27–87
Powdered chocolate drink	150ml cup	1–6
Chocolate milk drink	150ml cup	1–3
Chocolate bar	50g bar	5–36

(MAFF Food Safety Directorate. Survey of caffeine and other methylxanthines in energy drinks and other caffeine-containing products (Updated information). Food Surveillance Information Sheet 144, March 1998)

The stimulating effect of caffeine may even be helpful for those runners who struggle to run first thing in the morning. Runners who unwillingly have to include early-morning runs in their training programme may well find that drinking a cup of coffee on waking can help increase mental activity and alertness.

Studies suggest that an ergogenic effect can be achieved with dosages as low as 3mg per kg body weight, but that 6mg per kg body weight may be more effective at increasing free fatty acid mobilization. Even at 9mg per kg body weight, health risks are considered minimal. Some individuals are particularly sensitive to caffeine and for them even small doses can produce jitters and shakes. At doses above 9mg per kg body weight, some individuals experience stomach upsets.

Prior to January 2004, levels of urinary caffeine exceeding 12µg per ml resulted in a positive drug test but since that date caffeine has been removed completely from the World Anti-Doping Agency list of prohibited substances.

Using large doses of caffeine prior to the start or smaller doses of caffeine such as flat cola drinks in the later stages of endurance events is a practice that has been popular among professional cyclists for some time, and it certainly does appear to merit further investigation for marathon runners. Recent research has shown that a small dose of caffeine, about 1.5mg per kg body weight, in the last forty minutes of endurance exercise improved time-trial performance in the laboratory situation.

There have been concerns that caffeine has a diuretic effect and runners have been advised to avoid caffeine-containing drinks, even though there seems to be no support in the literature for such advice. What the literature does suggest is that large doses of caffeine (above 300mg) have an acute diuretic effect; that single caffeine doses at the levels found in tea, coffee, cola drinks and so on, have little or no diuretic effect and that regular caffeine users get used to the effects of caffeine, which then lessens its actions.

Caffeine is, therefore, relatively safe for healthy runners and is now totally legal. However, those runners who decide to use caffeine in a marathon must have practised and perfected the technique in long training runs.

CARNITINE (L-CARNITINE)

Carnitine is involved in both the transfer of fatty acids across the mitochondrial membrane, where they can be oxidized and used as a source of fuel, and in the oxidation of carbohydrate. It has therefore been suggested that carnitine supplementation may help to spare the limited supplies of muscle glycogen and therefore improve endurance performance. Carnitine is obtained from a diet that contains meat, milk and dairy products. It can also be made in the liver and kidneys from the amino acids lysine and methionine, so even runners adhering to a vegan diet are not at risk of developing a carnitine deficiency.

At present there does not appear to be enough scientific data to show that carnitine supplementation is effective in boosting energy supplies. It is therefore unlikely that taking extra carnitine as a supplement will be of any benefit to an endurance runner.

Carnitine supplements are also sold on the basis that, as they increase fat oxidation, they must be effective in promoting weight loss, although evidence is somewhat lacking. Many slimming products that contain carnitine also contain other ingredients, including ephedrine, which is on the WADA list of prohibited substances. Any runner who is tempted to test out the ergogenic effects of carnitine must avoid using D- and DL-carnitine supplements, as they can produce harmful effects in the body. L-carnitine is both safe and legal, although not necessarily effective.

COENZYME Q10

Coenzyme Q10 (CoQ10) is a naturally occurring fat-soluble substance that is involved in the generation of ATP in the mitochondria of all tissues. It also functions as an antioxidant, removing free radicals from the circulation and moderating lipid peroxidation. Much of the research has studied the effects of CoQ10 in heart patients, where improvements have been noted in heart function, VO_2max and exercise performance, but published studies where supplements have been given to healthy athletes have shown no such positive effects. As far as the antioxidant effects are concerned, money would be better spent on buying fresh fruit and vegetables on a regular basis. CoQ10 is legal and appears to be safe in doses of 100 to 150mg, but it is ineffective as an ergogenic supplement.

CREATINE

Creatine is a naturally occurring compound found in meat and fish. The diet supplies about 1g per day for meat-eating individuals (1kg of fresh steak contains approximately 5g of creatine), the remainder being synthesized in the liver, pancreas and kidneys and other tissues from the amino acids arginine, methionine and glycine. In normal healthy individuals, muscle creatine is broken down, at the rate of 2g per day, to creatinine, which passes freely into the circulation and is then excreted by the kidneys. Creatine supplementation causes a marked and rapid rise in creatine phosphate levels in muscle. This is of particular benefit to those involved in power/speed sports, which are dependent on the ATP-CP energy system to fuel high-intensity, short-duration, short-recovery training sessions. Creatine supplementation does not appear to enhance running performance, which is not surprising, as the contribution from the ATP-CP energy system is minimal (*see* Chapter 1). Indeed, creatine supplementation results in an increase in body mass, which may have a detrimental effect on running performance.

There appear to be no reasons to doubt the safety of creatine when an appropriate dosage is used. It is also legal, although individual national governing bodies of sport may ban it, as the French Rugby Union has done. Those who are curious to know more about creatine are referred to The American College of Sports Medicine consensus statement on creatine. (The American College of Sports Medicine Roundtable on the physiological and health effects of oral creatine supplementation. *Med. Sci. Sports Exerc.*, Vol 32, No.3, pp.706–717, 2000.)

GLYCEROL

Glycerol is found naturally in many foods and is also manufactured by the hydrolysis of fats for use in food products and cough medicines. When consumed with water it is absorbed rapidly and distributed quickly throughout the body, where it exerts an osmotic effect. The body retains the water drunk with it more effectively than water alone. In theory, hyperhydration with glycerol before and rehydration with glycerol during training and races in hot, humid conditions could be used to minimize dehydration in runners. Studies on the effects of glycerol on thermoregulation and performance have been mixed, however. Although drinking a glycerol solution does increase total body water, it is much less clear whether it actually enhances performance. More research is needed to establish whether glycerol increases intracellular fluid or whether it boosts circulation. Current evidence suggests it may be of value where heavy fluid losses are anticipated and dehydration is unavoidable, for example, during marathons in hot and humid conditions.

When diluted correctly, glycerol supplementation appears to be safe, although side-effects such as headaches, light-headedness, bloating, nausea and stomach upsets have been observed. Runners with medical conditions such as high blood pressure, diabetes, migraine and kidney problems must consult their doctor about the suitability and safety of using glycerol. Runners who are competing in a marathon where the conditions are expected to be hot need to practise using glycerol before the marathon in order to get the dosage right, to ensure there are no side-effects and to make sure that performance is not affected by the extra body weight caused by the water loading. Glycerol is legal, although it is considered by some to be unethical.

Proper hydration is vital for runners in training and races and dehydration can be avoided or at least minimized by the sensible use of sports drinks. These drinks not only supply fluid rapidly but top up diminishing carbohydrate supplies as well.

LOSS OF EXCESS BODY FAT

For many non-elite runners, loss of excess body fat is probably the safest and most effective way of improving performance (and health). Loss of body fat can make a significant difference to energy efficiency, as less weight needs to be moved along. Although the body needs some body fat, too much fat can best be described as 'excess baggage'. Running a marathon with a couple of bags of heavy shopping on each arm would definitely be very hard work! It has been suggested that a 72kg male runner could improve his marathon running time by approximately six minutes if he lost 5 per cent of his body weight – just 3.6kg (8lb). In fact, many runners who take up running initially to lose weight and to get fitter eventually end up running marathons.

THE BOTTOM LINE

Runners should seek advice from a qualified medical practitioner, accredited sports dietitian and/or registered nutritionist if they are in any doubt about the efficacy and safety of a supplement product. This can be through individual contact and consultation or through one of the respected running magazines, which have panels of experts to answer reader letters (*see* Appendix II). Some runners may find a particular nutritional supplement helpful but none will take the place of a well-planned training programme, adequate rest and recovery time, and the right running shoes and clothing – and certainly not the optimal diet for training and races.

CHAPTER 6
Special Considerations

Many runners will need to adapt the advice in previous chapters to meet their own more specific requirements including vegetarian, female, veteran, diabetic and disabled runners. The conditions in which the marathon is run, such as an excessively hot or cold climate, will also require certain adaptations to be made.

VEGETARIAN RUNNERS

The term 'vegetarian' covers a wide variety of diets that are followed for many reasons, including religion, culture, concern for animals and the environment, and health. Runners may also decide to become vegetarian as a way of increasing carbohydrate intake or because of weight issues. In a very small number of cases, following a vegetarian diet can be the start of disordered eating, which in time may lead to a full-blown eating disorder. For instance, a runner may start by omitting red meat, and respond to a perception of feeling better and experiencing some weight loss by omitting other foods. As more and more foods are removed from the diet, such runners put themselves at greater risk of becoming anorexic or bulimic, or at the very least too thin to run at their best.

It is unclear whether a vegetarian diet has any performance benefits over a non-vegetarian diet. Most importantly, the overall balance and variety of the diet must meet all the nutritional requirements for health and running performance. A vegetarian diet that is adequate in energy and protein, high in carbohydrate and low in fat, and provides all the other essential nutrients, is certainly better than a non-vegetarian diet containing large amounts of protein and fat with minimal carbohydrate (the Atkins diet, for example). However, as the vegetarian diet becomes stricter and more and more foods are omitted from the daily diet, greater care is needed to ensure that training is supported by the complete range of essential nutrients, and enough of the right sort of energy.

Differences in Vegetarian Diets

Semi- or Demi-Vegetarians

Exclude red meat but eat poultry, game, fish, dairy foods and eggs. Red meat may be avoided for ethical reasons or because of concern about the safety of meat. Nutritionally, the diet could be lacking in iron.

Pesco-Vegetarians

Eat fish, dairy foods and eggs but no red meat, poultry or game. Nutrients that might be lacking are iron and zinc. However, if plenty of shellfish and oily fish are eaten regularly, zinc requirements should be met.

Lacto-Ovo-Vegetarians

Eat dairy products and eggs but no meat, poultry, game or fish, or ingredients derived from them, such as gelatine or rennet. Nutrients that may be lacking are iron, zinc and possibly essential fatty acids. Lean meat is a good source of omega-6 fatty acids and oily fish a good source of omega-3 fatty acids. Excluding these sources places a much heavier reliance on the use of vegetable oils, although including eggs that have been laid by hens fed a diet rich in omega-3 fatty acids will certainly make a valuable contribution. Some lacto-ovo vegetarians rely on large amounts of milk and cheese to meet their protein requirements; this can lead to consumption of unhealthy amounts of total and saturated fat. Including low-fat milk, cheese and yoghurt, together with eggs, in the daily diet will ensure that the diet contains sufficient protein as well as the full complement of essential amino acids.

Lacto-Vegetarians

Eat dairy foods but no eggs or animal flesh. Again, iron, zinc and essential fatty acids may be lacking.

Ovo-Vegetarians

Eat eggs as their only animal product. Avoidance of dairy products, the best source of calcium, means that other sources of calcium must be included in the diet on a daily basis and in plentiful amounts. Controversy continues about the acceptable number of eggs that can be consumed in a week. The general consensus is no more than four, but the World Health Organization suggests an upper limit of ten eggs a week from all sources. As saturated fat intake from other sources will be low in this type of diet, it seems reasonable for ovo-vegetarians to follow the WHO guidelines if they wish. Regular physical activity is recommended as part of a healthy lifestyle to help keep cholesterol levels and blood pressure down and to prevent overweight and obesity. Runners will therefore already be reducing these risks by following a weekly training programme. Although eggs are a rich source of cholesterol, the greater health concern is not about dietary cholesterol itself but the cholesterol that is made in the body from dietary saturated fats. The high intake of cholesterol from eggs is only a concern to those who already have a high cholesterol level. Again, careful choice of foods will be necessary to ensure adequate intakes of iron, zinc and essential fatty acids. Eating up to ten omega-3-enriched eggs a week will certainly meet requirements for these essential fatty acids.

Vegans

Eat no animal products, relying solely on plant-based foods such as cereals, fruit, vegetables, nuts and seeds. Many manufactured foods will also be avoided, as additives such as emulsifiers are often of animal origin. Information about additives in foods can be obtained directly from the manufacturer (contact details will be on the packaging) or the Vegetarian Society (see Appendix II). In the vegan diet, protein requirements will be met if the overall diet contains enough energy. Inclusion of a wide variety of cereals, pulses and green vegetable sources will ensure the correct mix of amino acids. Current thinking is that the balance of amino acids must be achieved on a daily basis but that it is no longer considered necessary to achieve this at each meal. Other nutrients that can be lacking in a vegan diet are vitamin B_{12}, iron, zinc, calcium, essential fatty acids and vitamin B_2.

Fruitarians

Eat nothing but raw or dried fruit, nuts, seeds, honey and olive oil. Such a diet cannot meet nutritional requirements and will not support a marathon training programme effectively.

Macrobiotic Diets

Progress through seven levels, starting with what is mainly a vegetarian diet (which may contain fish) and eventually reaching the most extreme level, now seldom followed, which contains just brown rice. With careful planning, the less extreme levels of the diet would support marathon training. However, progression through the levels would make it harder and eventually totally impossible to train. Indeed, there have been several deaths as a result of living on brown rice alone because such a diet is totally lacking in many of the essential nutrients.

Practical Issues

Vegetarians generally consume more carbohydrate than non-vegetarians because of the greater reliance on grains, pulses, fruits and vegetables. However, care must be taken to make sure that sufficient and varied sources of protein are included at all meals. Some vegetarian meals can take time to prepare and cook, so it is a good idea to keep a stock of canned beans of different types, chickpeas and lentils for emergencies, or when a meal needs to be put together quickly, for example, after an evening training run. There is no shortage of vegetarian cookery books and those that give preparation and cooking times can be particularly useful. Many meat recipes, such as Bolognese sauces and shepherd's pie, can be adapted fairly easily by substituting meat mince with canned or dried lentils, soya or Quorn mince. Tofu can be used instead of chicken in other recipes such as stir-fries, casseroles and pasta bakes.

USEFUL VEGETARIAN SOURCES OF NUTRIENTS

(Items in brackets will not be suitable for all categories of vegetarianism.)

Protein: beans, peas, lentils, Quorn, tofu, soya, soya milk, nuts, seeds and cereals and cereal products. (Milk and dairy products.)

Iron: wholegrain cereals, fortified breakfast cereals, beans, peas, lentils, dark green leafy vegetables, dried fruit, nuts and seeds. (Shellfish and egg yolks.)

Zinc: wholegrain cereals, bread, beans, peas, lentils, nuts and seeds. (Shellfish, milk and dairy products and eggs.)

Calcium: soya milk and soya products fortified with calcium, sesame seeds and tahini paste, dark green leafy vegetables, oranges, almonds, Brazil nuts, peanuts and peanut butter, almonds, beans, peas and lentils, white flour and bread that is fortified, hard water. (Canned fish, but only if the bones are eaten, milk and dairy products.)

Vitamin B_{12}: fortified foods including breakfast cereals, yeast extracts, soya products, fermented soya foods such as miso – a bean paste/sauce and tempeh or soybean cake, supplements. (Milk, dairy products and eggs.)

FEMALE RUNNERS

Female runners tend to be smaller, carry more body fat and have less muscle mass than male runners. Excessive body fat is counter-productive to endurance running and some female runners will want to reduce it. This will be recommended for some, but not all female runners who embark on a diet aiming to lose weight or body fat actually need to. Significant numbers of women are constantly trying to lose weight by a variety of dieting methods, so it is not surprising that many female runners are not happy with their weight, shape and body-fat levels.

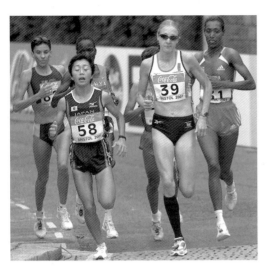

Paula Radcliffe (*front right*) in action at the World Half Marathon in Bristol. (EMPICS)

DIFFERENCES BETWEEN THE SEXES

Females have a higher body fat content.

Females generally have lower maximum cardiac outputs and lower stroke volumes.

Blood volume tends to be lower in females.

Males have about 10 per cent more haemoglobin than females.

Males achieve higher VO_2max values.

Females burn fat at a higher rate than males, which has a glycogen-sparing effect and limits feelings of fatigue.

Oestrogen can increase the force of muscular contractions during endurance exercise so the body can work harder.

As race distances increase, females tend to slow down less than males.

Females have a menstrual cycle.

It is worth emphasizing the fact that women are supposed to have more fat than men because of the key role that body fat plays in reproduction. Excessive reduction in body-fat levels can lead to a variety of problems that not only affect running performance but can also result in serious health problems.

Menstrual Matters

Throughout the fertile stage of a female's life, hormonal changes control cyclical changes in the reproductive organs. Every month, an egg is released from the ovaries and the lining of the uterus or womb thickens in readiness to accept a fertilized egg. If fertilization does not happen, the lining is discarded and a menstrual bleed, or period, occurs.

The menstrual cycle can affect running performance and, although it may not be possible to ensure that marathons are run at the 'best' time in the cycle, at least it is reassuring to know why it may feel tougher one week compared with another. Women tend to run faster before ovulation (the follicular phase)

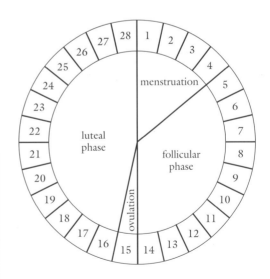

The menstrual cycle.

but less well between ovulation and the next period (the luteal phase). During the luteal phase, ventilation rate increases and running feels harder. This is because perceived effort is closely related to the depth and frequency of breathing. During the luteal phase, both running economy and mental vigour or strength of mind are reduced. Runners can feel rather miserable and tired during this phase, which can also make running feel that much harder. However, running does release endorphins, which have a feel-good effect and some females who normally experience painful periods often find that running during their period can actually minimize discomfort.

Some studies have suggested that females are more responsive to carbohydrate loading during the follicular phase of the menstrual cycle, while others indicate that loading may be more efficient in the luteal phase. The obvious recommendation would be to carbohydrate load regardless of the stage in the menstrual cycle.

The menstrual cycle can be altered by use of the contraceptive pill. This is normally taken on a daily basis for twenty-one days, followed by seven days when the pill is not taken and a 'withdrawal bleed' occurs. With advice from her doctor, a runner may wish to continue to take the pill for longer in order to avoid a bleed around the time of a marathon. The pill can also be helpful for runners who experience painful and very heavy periods. It has been suggested that the contraceptive pill may reduce aerobic capacity and therefore affect performance, which adds another factor into the debate. Runners in doubt about changing their medication should consult their own doctor. Female runners are particularly at risk of poor iron status because of iron losses during menstruation. This may be compounded by a poor dietary intake and losses through sweating and foot strike haemolysis. Particular attention must be paid to practical ways of increasing iron intake (*see* Chapter 2).

Pregnancy

Pregnancy is not the time to start training for a marathon. In fact, one of the main reasons why runners withdraw from races is because they (or their partner) are pregnant. Although running should not be taken up after becoming pregnant, there is no reason why pregnant runners should not continue some running, as long as there are no problems and the pregnancy is progressing well. In published studies of exercise throughout pregnancy, women who averaged 2.5–4km (1.5–2.5 miles) per day had no apparent harmful effects. Studies have in any case shown a voluntary reduction in mileage during pregnancy. There are some potential concerns about exercise in pregnancy, the major one being that physical activity can raise maternal core temperature, which in turn can raise fetal temperature. The recommendation is therefore to ensure that maternal temperature does not rise above 38°C.

Experts consider that, as energy is used more efficiently during pregnancy and because there may also be a reduction in energy expenditure, it is only necessary to increase energy intake in the last trimester of pregnancy (twenty-six to forty weeks), by an extra 200kcal a day. A pregnant runner will obviously require more energy than a non-pregnant runner in the first and second trimesters because of the energy cost of running. However, energy intake should not be greater than the energy intake before pregnancy and, indeed, as the pregnancy advances and mileage is cut back, intake may need to be lowered until the third trimester. Monitoring of body weight, along with other routine pregnancy checks, will establish if the right amount of food is being consumed. Carbohydrate intake must also be maintained, as pregnant females use more carbohydrate both at rest and during exercise than non-pregnant females.

SAFETY CONSIDERATIONS FOR EXERCISING WHEN PREGNANT

Avoid prolonged or strenuous exercise in the first trimester. (Volume and intensity will certainly drop off automatically in the second trimester.)

Maintain adequate nutrition and hydration, paying particular attention to fluid intake before, during and after exercise. Keep a check on urine colour, volume and frequency. Use pre- and post-running weighing to check fluid losses through sweating.

Avoid exercising in warm and/or humid conditions.

Pay attention to warming up and cooling down because joints and connective tissue, particularly in the pelvic region, become 'looser' as pregnancy progresses.

Avoid rigid training programmes, adopting instead a flexible programme that takes account of increasing weight, change in body shape and overall feelings and attitude towards training.

Switch to other forms of exercise as running becomes harder and less enjoyable. Walking and swimming are excellent alternatives, particularly during the later stages of pregnancy.

POSSIBLE CAUSES OF MENSTRUAL DYSFUNCTION

Reduction in energy intake.

Increase in training volume.

More commonly both a reduction in energy intake and an increase in training volume.

Reduction in body weight and body fat composition.

Restricted food choices and poor eating habits.

After the birth, running can be introduced gradually, as long as the medical staff in charge of the post-natal check-up are happy that it is both physically and medically safe.

Menstrual Dysfunction

Some female runners training hard for a marathon find that their periods stop or at least that their menstrual cycle becomes irregular, particularly as they increase their weekly mileage. Loss of periods occurs much more when women are running 130km (80 miles) or more a week compared with those who are only running 30km (20 miles) a week. However, stepping up the mileage is rarely the only cause. Menstrual dysfunction can be a cause for concern because the reduced levels of female hormones can lead to a bone-health threat, which, in turn, may be linked to an increase in sports-related injuries and development of osteoporosis. Together with the disruption to the menstrual cycle and possible increase in frequency of injuries, the runner may become more fatigued and irritable. Overall, running will certainly not be going well at this stage.

When body fat falls to a very low level, periods stop. This is nature's way of protecting against the occurrence of a pregnancy that the body would not be capable of supporting. A reduction in body-fat composition is therefore linked to either amenorrhoea (loss of periods) or oligomenorrhoea (infrequent periods).

The most important trigger is a negative energy balance. An intake of fewer than 1,800kcal a day is unlikely to meet the energy demands of a marathon training programme and, depending on the foods eaten, may not meet requirements for carbohydrate, protein, vitamins and minerals, either. Female runners need to place less importance on body weight and the reading on the bathroom scales, and focus more on food choices, meal patterns, when and how much food is being eaten, and how their training programme is progressing. Meals should never be missed and time should always be made to have breakfast every day. Eating enough to kick-start the menstrual cycle may mean eating 20 per cent more than is needed to maintain body weight.

Increased intake should centre round carbohydrates, fruit and vegetables and moderate but not excessive intakes of protein rather than fat. Runners in doubt that their diet provides all the essential vitamins and minerals on a daily basis should include a one-a-day multivitamin and mineral supplement, but avoid taking an assortment of single vitamins and minerals unless advised otherwise by a medically or nutritionally qualified person. Once a healthy weight has been achieved, and continues to be maintained as mileage increases, such a supplement will probably no longer be needed, particularly if a wide variety of foods from all the main food groups is being enjoyed on a daily basis.

Bones

Bone is an active tissue that is constantly being broken down and built up again. When breakdown is occurring faster than build-up, there is a reduction in bone mineral density (BMD), which leads to the development of the disease osteoporosis. The amount of bone per unit volume is reduced, although there is no change in the composition of the bone tissue itself. The bone becomes porous and brittle, and fractures easily – osteoporosis is often called the 'brittle bone disease'. It is also sometimes referred to as the 'silent disease', as there are no obvious symptoms until fractures

occur. Around 70,000 hip fractures occur in British women each year and, indeed, female osteoporosis has been estimated to cost the National Health Service in the UK almost £750 million a year.

Bone density in runners tends to be higher than in the sedentary population, particularly in the parts of the skeleton that are stressed during running – calcaneum (heel bone), tibia (shin bone), femur (thigh bone) and spine. However, amenorrhoeic runners with low body-fat levels and low levels of circulating oestrogen behave rather like post-menopausal women. They experience accelerated bone loss, resulting in reduced bone density, and this in

---

BONE MINERAL DENSITY IN FEMALES

Increases during adolescence and early adult life, adolescence being a particularly critical period, when approximately 40 per cent of peak bone mass (PBM) is laid down.

By twenty years of age, 90 to 95 per cent of PBM is reached.

Skeleton is at its strongest at thirty to thirty-five years of age.

Slow, age-related decline starts after thirty years of age.

Additional accelerated loss at the time of the menopause lasts five to eight years.

Higher PBM can delay onset of osteoporosis, in other words, the amount of bone in the elderly skeleton is determined by the amount present at maturity and by the rate of subsequent bone loss.

Bone mineral density of the lower body in female distance runners develops at the expense of bone in the upper body.

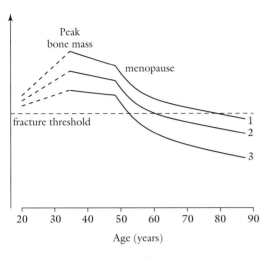

1 Normal menstrual cycle with regular exercise
2 Normal menstrual cycle
3 Long-term amenorrhoea

Changes in bone density with age.

turn puts them at greater risk of suffering a traumatic or stress fracture. Even if bone density does not fall so low that stress fractures occur, there are long-term health implications. Young women who are losing bone when they should still be accumulating it will have a lower peak bone mass in mid-adulthood and this will inevitably increase the risk of osteoporosis and fractures in later adulthood.

Dietary calcium plays a role in determining BMD and, although its main effect occurs during childhood and adolescence, it is important that female runners maintain a calcium intake to meet their requirement of 700mg a day. For runners who are amenorrhoeic or oligomenorrhoeic, intakes should be increased to 1,500mg, usually by a combination of diet and the use of a sensible supplement. Recent evidence suggests that milk and dairy products may confer an additional benefit, besides their excellent calcium content. Fruit and vegetables may also play a protective role. Contrary to advice that is often given, moderate intakes of caffeine appear to have no significant effect on calcium balance and bone mass. High intakes of caffeine are only likely to exacerbate the risk of osteoporosis if calcium intake is already low. Heavy and regular alcohol intake is associated with a reduction in BMD and increased risk of fractures. Excessive amounts of protein should be avoided as, although protein in the diet increases calcium absorption, it also enhances urinary excretion so that there is a net reduction in the amount of calcium available. Including some resistance training into the overall marathon programme for the upper body as well as the lower body can also be beneficial. Not only can it boost muscle strength and add some body weight, primarily as useful muscle rather than as body fat, but it can also improve BMD.

Bone loss can occur quickly in the young female runner who has stopped having periods and she should be encouraged to seek advice and treatment from her doctor as soon as possible. Treatment of amenorrhoea aims to prevent bone loss and to re-establish a normal menstrual cycle. The latter can take time, which may not be what the runner has in terms of her bones, particularly if she has been amenorrhoeic for some time. In this case, the likely treatment will be the use of hormone therapy to boost the level of circulating oestrogen. Changes in lifestyle will take longer and will, of course, need the cooperation of the runner. The runner should be encouraged to decrease training activity by 10 to 20 per cent and increase energy intake to ensure a weight gain of 2 to 3 per cent of current body weight. Calcium intake should be increased to 1,500mg per day and resistance training used to boost muscle strength and help bone mineralization. The runner should be encouraged to consult a sports dietitian for help with her diet (*see* Appendix I for contact details of DISEN).

Eating Disorders

A marathon training programme needs to be supported by a diet that provides energy, nutrients and fluids in the required amounts for the runner. Unfortunately, many female runners believe that cutting back food intake and losing weight will improve running (as well as appearance). For some runners, a reduction in body fat may well lead to improved running times, but this can be carried too far, with not only a loss in performance but serious health implications.

ADVERSE EFFECTS OF UNNECESSARY WEIGHT LOSS ON RUNNING PERFORMANCE

Loss of muscle tissue.

Low glycogen stores.

Dehydration and electrolyte imbalance (restricted intake and, for some, losses through vomiting and use of laxatives), affecting coordination, balance and muscle function.

Long-term effects may include increased susceptibility to stress fractures, loss of periods and premature osteoporosis.

Initial changes in eating habits can happen almost without family and friends noticing. By the time others are aware that there is something wrong, the runner may already be suffering to some degree from an eating disorder. Eating disorders are more prevalent among females, but males are also at risk, especially if they are involved in a sport – for example, distance running, lightweight rowing and horse-racing – where a low level of body fat is considered a benefit. A runner might initially follow a vegetarian diet as a perfectly acceptable way of limiting food choices. She might then adopt a more irregular eating pattern by avoiding certain meals or by putting off the first meal or snack of the day for as long as possible. Other people might notice her drinking much greater volumes of fluid (to feel full), or snacking on 'bad' or 'forbidden' foods. She may become more and more selective about foods she does eat and give the impression that she is scared of anything that contains even the smallest amount of fat. Carbohydrate-containing foods may then become the next group to be excluded. Some runners may feel guilty when they feel full or have eaten what they perceive to be a lot of food, while others may get panicky about food and eat very quickly. Vomiting after eating will then be the obvious answer for many.

The diagnostic criteria according to the Diagnostic and Statistical Manual of Mental Disorders (DSM-IV TR) for Anorexia Nervosa and Bulimia Nervosa include both physical and psychological observations. A list of behavioural warning signs is also given, many of which could be picked up by family, friends or other runners. Physiotherapists and doctors who treat runners with injuries may well notice warning signs too.

Diagnosis and Help

Some runners will eventually be diagnosed with a clinical eating disorder according to the strict criteria in the DSM-IV TR, published in 2000. Others will present with less severe or sub-clinical forms of eating disorders but still showing many of the symptoms described. They may restrict food intake but not enough to be diagnosed as anorexic. They may binge and purge but not regularly enough to be diagnosed as bulimic. Many of the traits they display (high achievement, obsessive behaviour, perfectionism) are common and,

BEHAVIOURAL WARNING SIGNS IN EATING DISORDERS

Behavioural warning signs in anorexia
Obsessed with fat grams and/or calories.
Wears baggy clothes to disguise thinness.
Always dieting.
Dislikes eating in public or with friends, grows anxious around food.
Gives suspicious reasons for not eating ('I already ate', 'I'm feeling sick', and so on).
Indulges in peculiar eating rituals, chewing foods excessively, cutting food into tiny pieces.
Exercises despite injuries and against advice.
Panics if food or exercise routine is interrupted; inflexible.
Reads all food labels.
Becomes a vegetarian or gives up most perceived high-fat animal products.
Drinks excessive amount of water or diet soda.
Depression.
Social withdrawal.
Weighs self multiple times daily.
Complains of feeling cold.
Overly 'self-less' to the point of denying right to eat.
Dissatisfaction with body.
Fear of gaining fat despite appearing emaciated.
Perfectionist.
Extreme fear of failure or criticism.
Emotionally or sexually inhibited.
Obsessive/compulsive.

Behavioural warning signs in bulimia
Does not gain weight despite eating large quantities.
Goes to the bathroom immediately after eating.
Watery eyes, sniffing after bathroom trips.
Appears to take multiple showers daily (to cover sound of vomiting).
Dislikes eating in public or with friends, grows anxious around food.
Exercises despite injuries and against advice.
Panics if food or exercise routine is interrupted; inflexible.
Reads all food labels.
Becomes a vegetarian or gives up most perceived high-fat animal products.
Drinks excessive amount of water or diet soda.
Depression.
Social withdrawal.
Weighs self multiple times daily.
Carries breath mints or tooth-care products.
Hiding food.
Evidence of eating large amounts of food in secret.
Weight change.
Depression, mood swings or isolation.
Perfectionist.
Fearful of abandonment.
Hypochondriac.
Temper tantrums.

(Courtesy Beth Glace MS, Sports Nutritionist, Nicholas Institute of Sports Medicine and Athletic Trauma)

indeed, expected and often essential in the competitive sporting world. This form of sub-clinical eating disorder is referred to as 'anorexia athletica'.

It is not easy for a runner with an eating disorder to get better by herself and invariably professional help and support will be needed. A runner who accepts that she has an eating problem, and acknowledges that she needs help, will have taken one of the hardest steps towards recovery. The next step is to find someone she can trust, perhaps a friend, parent or fellow runner, with whom she can discuss it. The Eating Disorders Association has a helpline for strictly confidential calls, as well as a list of counsellors who can offer help (*see* Appendix II). A runner's local GP will be able to carry out a medical assessment and possibly provide treatment or, alternatively, a referral to a specialist.

DSM-IV TR DIAGNOSTIC CRITERIA FOR
ANOREXIA NERVOSA AND BULIMIA NERVOSA

Anorexia Nervosa (DSM-IV 307.1)
Refusal to maintain weight at or above 85 per cent of that expected.
Intense fear of gaining weight or becoming fat.
Distorted body image or denial of seriousness of current low body weight.
Amenorrhea: lack of three consecutive cycles.
Specific types
Restricting Type: not regularly engaging in binge-eating or purging behaviour.
Binge-Eating/Purging Type: regularly engaging in binge-eating or purging behaviour.

Bulima (DSM-IV 307.51)
Recurrent episodes of binge-eating:
Eating in a discrete period of time considerably more than the average person.

Lack of control during eating session.
Recurrent inappropriate compensatory behaviour:
Self-induced vomiting, laxatives, emetics, diuretics, fasting or excess exercise.
Bingeing and compensatory behaviours occuring on average at least twice-weekly for three months.
Self-image unduly based upon body shape and weight.
Does not occur exclusively during anorexia nervosa.
Specific types
Purging Type: regularly engaging in self-induced vomiting, misuse of laxatives, diuretics, enemas.
Non-Purging Type: using other compensatory behaviours such as fasting or excessive exercise.

VETERANS

'Age is not a barrier to performance, only an inconvenience' (Darrell Meard, *Oxford Textbook of Sports Medicine*, 1994). The official age for a Veteran in distance running (or Master, as they are known in the USA) is thirty-five for women and forty for men, which is, of course, relatively young. Such athletes may not be concerned by special issues, but there may be specific considerations to take into account for the more elderly runner.

The older runner may be an athlete who has run from an early age, perhaps extending event distances with time. Alternatively, he or she may have decided to take up running late in life for a variety of reasons, including weight loss or prevention of weight gain, to stay or get physically fit, to reduce the risk of developing coronary heart disease or high blood pressure, for enjoyment, to raise money for charity, or even for a bet!

If physical activity levels are kept up through regular running, a greater lean body mass will be maintained. The veteran runner will be able to enjoy eating more food than his or her sedentary contemporaries, while keeping a healthy body weight. By selecting a wide variety of foods from the basic food groups, and following the advice in Chapters 2 and 3, veteran runners should have no problem in meeting requirements for both health and running. Including some appropriate strength training as part of the marathon programme will help to maintain muscle mass. Including oily fish regularly in the diet or, alternatively, taking a daily supplement of cod liver oil will help to protect and relieve joints that are beginning to

ANTI-AGEING EFFECTS OF RUNNING

Prevention of muscle wastage and maintenance of lean body mass.

Maintenance of muscle strength.

Maintenance of bone density and prevention/delay of onset of osteoporosis.

Protecting the cardiovascular system by making the arteries more elastic and efficient.

Improving efficiency of the heart and circulation. Regular physical activity can halve the risk of developing coronary heart disease and help to reduce blood pressure.

Improve serum lipid profiles by reducing total cholesterol and raising HDL cholesterol.

become problematic. Research has shown that older runners can tolerate moderate amounts of exercise without accelerating development of osteoarthritis.

The veteran runner does need to address some age-related aspects of the diet. Dehydration and heat-related injuries are a greater risk for the veteran than for the younger runner. Renal function is lowered and there is a decreased ability to concentrate urine. This can lead to an impaired ability to maintain body temperature during exercise in hot or humid conditions. Heat intolerance in the aged seems to be related primarily to the decrease in physical fitness observed in the vast majority of older individuals. The fit veteran runner will have a greater tolerance to exercise in the heat than those of a similar age who lead a sedentary lifestyle. However, the thirst sensation tends to decrease with age in everyone. Research has shown that active healthy men aged sixty-seven to seventy-five years of age were less thirsty and voluntarily drank less water when water-deprived for twenty-four hours than similarly deprived men aged twenty to thirty-one years. The sweat response to exercise is also reduced with age but this is not so marked in those who run on a regular basis. It is vital, therefore, that, as veteran runners become progressively more veteran, they monitor their fluid intake on a regular basis. Advice already given in Chapter 3 applies equally to the veteran marathon runner in both training and races – to hydrate well before running, to start drinking before the thirst mechanism kicks in during running, and to continue drinking once running has ceased, until totally hydrated again.

When runners have the choice, they should avoid the hottest times of the day and, whenever they can, they should try to run in the shade rather than out in the glare of the sun. Light-coloured running gear and a sensible, practical hat can also help to reduce the risk of heat stress. All runners should take heed of muscle cramps, cool dry skin, a faster pulse, any sickness, thirst or overwhelming tiredness, as these can all be indicators of heat stress.

THE DIABETIC RUNNER

Diabetes mellitus is one of the most common chronic diseases, affecting about 1.4 million people in the UK, with the number expected to reach three million by 2010. Diabetics do not have enough insulin, a hormone normally produced by the pancreas, which is responsible for the transfer of glucose from the blood to the tissues. There are two types of diabetes. In Type 1 diabetes, the body either does not produce any insulin or it does not produce enough. The reasons why this should happen are poorly understood. Type 1 diabetics will require treatment with insulin for the rest of their lives. Type 2 diabetes is an insulin-resistant form, where either insulin is produced but in insufficient amounts,

BENEFITS OF EXERCISE FOR PEOPLE WITH DIABETES

Improves insulin sensitivity so that less insulin is needed to maintain normal blood-sugar levels.

Cardiovascular risk factors are decreased as HDL cholesterol (the beneficial type) levels rise and LDL cholesterol (the harmful type) levels fall.

Muscle mass is increased and body fat is reduced, both of which help to improve insulin sensitivity.

or it is produced in an ineffective form. Among Type 2 diabetics, 80 per cent are overweight and, as the incidence of obesity rises, more people are developing this type of diabetes at a younger age than in the past. Diet and lifestyle changes, such as a reduction in energy intake and an increase in physical activity, are often all that is needed to treat this type of diabetes. Some people with Type 2 diabetes do need treatment with oral hypoglycaemic drugs, to increase insulin production or to make the insulin that is produced more effective, while others will actually need insulin medication. Diabetics constantly have to work at keeping their blood-sugar levels within the normal range. Adding exercise into the equation can be a real challenge for a diabetic, particularly a newly diagnosed one, and yet exercise can provide important benefits to people with diabetes.

During exercise, contracting muscles have an insulin-like effect as they take up glucose from the blood. In the non-diabetic there is a fall in insulin production, which prevents hypoglycaemia (low blood sugar). Type 1 diabetics and Type 2 diabetics using insulin will need to adjust pre-exercise insulin dosage and carbohydrate intake before, during and after exercise, to avoid becoming hypoglycaemic. There are

many variables that will affect diabetic control in relation to running and, more specifically, training for and running in a marathon. It is therefore impossible to produce recommendations or a set of guidelines that will apply to all diabetic runners. However, a number of general points can be made.

All first-time runners or those who have never undertaken distance running should consult their doctor or consultant to make sure there are no contraindications. Clothing needs to be suitable and special attention must be paid to footwear. A bumbag can be used to carry any testing equipment, glucose tablets, drinks and a card containing contact details and advice about dealing with a hypoglycaemic attack. Runners should always wear an SOS bracelet and make sure that someone knows where they are going to be running. Joining a running club may be the best way to ensure 'safe running'. Diabetic runners would do well to follow the example of elite runners and keep a training log. This will help to make sure that diet and insulin dosages match the training and races. Once three or more training runs are being done every week, overall insulin requirements will fall by 25 to 40 per cent. This does not include the reduction needed on running days but reflects the beneficial effects of exercise.

It is important to remember that exercise is always associated with extra energy consumption and that exercise stimulates glucose uptake into muscle cells. The same amount of insulin allows more glucose to be metabolized during exercise than when at rest. It is important to make insulin dose adjustments before exercise, and to be aware of the risk of hypoglycaemia and of the need to take on board extra carbohydrate to cover the increase in requirement.

Requirements for the diabetic runner will be unique to each individual and the ideal situation would involve a team comprising runner, endocrinologist, diabetic dietitian and sports dietitian. This team can work out the requirements and monitor and make adjustments as necessary through the marathon programme.

PRE- AND POST-MARATHON PLAN FOR THE DIABETIC RUNNER

Four days before the marathon
Taper training.
Carbohydrate load with 8–10g per kg body weight per day for three to four days, using foods with a low glycaemic index.

Pre-marathon meal
A meal taken two hours before the race for runners using ordinary soluble insulin. For those using a short-acting insulin analogue, the meal should be eaten one to one and a half hours before the race. It should be mainly carbohydrate and with a low glycaemic index. As a guide, aim for 2–4g carbohydrate per kg body weight.

Sports drinks with a carbohydrate content of 5 to 8 per cent can be used immediately before the race, particularly if there is a need to correct relative hypoglycaemia.

During the race
Sports drinks as above should be of benefit to diabetic runners but, as with non-diabetic runners, they must have been used in long training runs prior to the marathon itself.

After the race
Replacement of carbohydrate is probably most effectively achieved by the use of the sports drink used before and during the race, followed later by a large meal containing a high proportion of low-GI carbohydrate-rich foods.

Even with reductions of insulin dose and extra carbohydrate, there will still be a tendency to hypoglycaemia on the following morning. Insulin dose will need to be reduced and extra carbohydrate taken on board.

Further recommended reading includes Bill Burr and Dinesh Nagi (eds), *Exercise and Sport in Diabetes* (John Wiley & Sons Ltd, 1999, reprinted July 2002; ISBN 0-471-98496-5) and Sheri R. Colberg, *The Diabetic Athlete* (Human Kinetics, 2001; ISBN 0-7360-3271-1).

DISABLED MARATHONERS

The same basic training diet principles apply to the wheelchair athlete as to the able-bodied runner. Fatigue will still be caused by either insufficient carbohydrate in the diet to provide energy for the working muscles and/or dehydration. Spinal-cord-injured athletes may not sweat below the point of spinal lesion but there is evidence that the sweat rate above this point is higher than average. Sweat losses will still need to be replaced by fluid intake but in some cases other methods of cooling will be needed, including water sprays, fans and possibly cooling vests or collars.

Those who suffer from autonomic dysreflexia or kidney problems should check with their medical team and work out a fluid programme together. If possible, they should also work

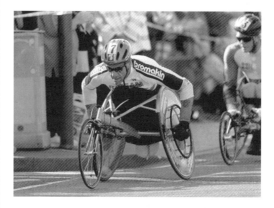

Wheelchair competitors in the London Marathon. (EMPICS)

with a sports dietitian who has experience of working with disabled athletes (*see* Appendix I for DISEN contact details).

The advice for blind and deaf runners will be no different from the advice for an able-bodied marathon runner.

COLD CLIMATES

Some marathons are run in cold countries, while others may take place on days that are unusually cold for the time of year. Such conditions may take runners by surprise if they have not prepared for running in such conditions. Runners should always check the weather forecast in the week leading up to a marathon. Normal body temperature is 37°C. In order to maintain this temperature in a cold environment, the body increases heat production by shivering and voluntary exercise, and by reducing the rate of heat loss by constricting the blood vessels to the skin, hands, feet and ears. Putting on more clothes will also help to reduce heat loss. If the conditions are very cold, core body temperature and VO_2max can fall, with a resulting loss in performance. In a moderately cold environment, however, endurance performance is actually enhanced.

Muscles that are well stocked with glycogen will not only supply energy for running but will also play a part in maintaining core body temperature, particularly in runners with relatively low body-fat stores. This is because carbohydrate is the main fuel for shivering. On cold-weather training runs lasting more than two hours, runners would do well to take a carbohydrate snack in a bum bag, as well as an appropriate sports drink. Runners tempted after a long run in the cold to warm up with a shot or two of alcohol should remember that alcohol dilates the blood vessels, which, in turn leads to an increase in the rate of heat loss. It would be practical and sensible to save the alcohol until fully hydrated.

When running in such conditions it is important to wear appropriate clothing, keep as dry as possible and maintain a high rate of heat production by exercising continuously. Multiple layers are recommended, with the layer next to the skin made of material that carries sweat away from the skin (polypropylene or cotton fishnet materials have a good wicking effect). Damp clothing increases the rate of heat loss from the body. Clothing should be adaptable, such as a zip front that can be undone and a hood that can be pulled up or pushed back off the head. The top layer of clothing should also be light, so that it can be easily carried if necessary. A lot of heat can be lost from the head, so some head cover should be worn.

Overall, the choice of clothing should be relative to the intensity of the exercise. It is also better to begin running feeling slightly cold, as a runner can soon over-heat if too many clothes are worn. A proper warm-up, continued right up to the start of the run, is vital. Wind can increase heat loss so, if possible, training runs should be started by going out facing the wind, when the cooling effect is greater but the runner is fresh and going at a good speed to generate some heat. Ideally, the latter part of the run, when the runner is tiring, pace is slowing up and heat production is dropping off, should be done with the back to the wind.

Runners should always run in populated areas when it is very cold and novice runners particularly should not be too ambitious about the distance they intend to cover, as it is important not to end up walking. At the end of the run, heat production will fall but heat loss will still be high, so to prevent hypothermia, extra layers of clothing should be put on and the runner should get into a warm environment as quickly as possible. Fingers, toes, ears and the face are all susceptible to frostbite as blood flow decreases. These areas should be checked regularly when out running for a long time in cold, windy conditions.

HOT CLIMATES

A sudden and unusual rise in temperature for the time of year may make a home marathon, scheduled to take place when weather conditions are usually ideal for running, a problem for the ill-prepared runner. Keeping a check on long- and short-range weather forecasts will help runners to be aware of any pending changes in conditions and allow them to make any necessary modifications to last-minute preparations. However, problems are more likely to occur when runners travel from a cool climate to take part in a marathon in a hot country. Problems may also occur when runners continue their training schedule during a holiday abroad. Training and competing in hotter and/or more humid conditions than a runner is used to will increase the risk of dehydration.

While away, runners can record fluid intake and urine habits and compare results to data collected while training at home (*see* Chapter 3). Hydration status can therefore be monitored and any necessary changes made to fluid intake to prevent or at least minimize dehydration. If feasible, regular weighing first thing every morning will help to indicate if there is progressive dehydration. However, weight loss may be due to eating less food in a hot environment. Runners should therefore assess for themselves whether they feel they are eating less. A comparison of fluid intake data and urine habits from home and data collected in the new environment should also help a runner ascertain if weight loss is due to dehydration rather than poor energy intake. Having identified the cause, the necessary actions can be taken to rectify things.

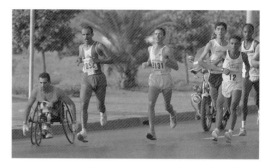

Wheelchair athletes and runners in the Marrakesh Marathon. (EMPICS)

If travel to the marathon involves a flight, a high fluid intake must be maintained throughout the travel time and there must be sufficient drinks in hand luggage to last until the final destination is reached. Room temperatures should not be set too low as constantly going from high to low temperatures can cause a sore throat, runny nose and cough. Leaving wet towels around the bedroom may seem untidy, but it can help to keep the atmosphere moist.

Heat Stroke

The decision to run a marathon in very hot and/or humid conditions should not be taken lightly. Without proper preparation for the marathon, and care on the day itself, runners can encounter serious health problems, culminating in heat stroke. In normally active healthy runners, the body's core temperature does not rise above 38°C. A slight rise above this temperature (moderate hyperthermia) will affect performance, but is unlikely to cause any major health problems. However, when there is complete failure of the body mechanisms that normally keep the core temperature within a healthy range, heat stroke can develop. This is a potentially life-threatening condition. The early warning signs – which runners should be aware of in themselves and in others – are irritability, confusion, apathy, belligerence, emotional instability and irrational behaviour. There may also be giddiness, undue fatigue and vomiting. Chills and goosebumps appear prior to the shutdown of skin circulation; once this happens, there is a much faster rise in core body temperature. The runner may start to hyperventilate and eventually there is a loss of coordination, the runner starts to stagger around, collapses, and can have a seizure, or lapse into a coma.

FACTORS THAT PRE-DISPOSE A RUNNER TO HEAT STROKE

Air temperature, humidity and wind movement – hot, humid, windless days reduce the amount of sweat evaporated from the skin so that body cooling is reduced.

Poor acclimatization (*see* pages 124–5).

Over-motivated or excessively keen runners who run too fast, too long (for example, the young, over-enthusiastic runner going for a personal best on a hot, humid day).

Dehydration.

Clothing that limits evaporation.

An excess of body fat. An overweight runner has to work harder than one with a healthier level of body fat. However, more muscle will generate more heat and a small, muscular runner may not have enough surface area to get rid of the excess heat.

Lack of fitness. Being aerobically fit has the same physiological advantages as heat acclimatization.

Recent feverishness or dehydration. Runners who have recently had illnesses such as an upper respiratory tract infection or gastroenteritis should not run in hot, humid conditions.

Practical Advice

Some runners will experience heat injuries during marathons run in high temperatures (above 23°C). At one end of the scale, these will result in heat exhaustion or fatigue and, at the other end, heat stroke. Runners with heat exhaustion usually have a normal body temperature but their pulse rate is faster, their skin is cold and sweaty, and they often feel drowsy and may vomit. Heat exhaustion responds to rest and cooling and can be prevented by adoption of a sensible fluid strategy.

Pre- and post-event cooling – by whole-body immersion or cold showers, use of cooling jackets or iced towels, or hand/feet cooling – can be achieved by applying the method for fifteen to thirty minutes. In fact, research has shown that hand cooling at 15 to 20°C is two to three times as effective as typical cooling jackets during pre- and post-event cooling. These strategies must be practised in training and never used for the first time in a race.

Other precautions include spongeing down or splashing the body with cool water whenever possible, using cooling fans, wearing minimal, light-coloured clothing that allows sweat to evaporate from the skin, starting out by running slowly and building up gradually to a comfortable speed, avoiding sprinting and being vigilant to the first symptoms of heat injury in oneself and in other runners – particularly headache, nausea, dizziness and poor co-ordination.

Races run in these conditions are definitely not the ones that runners should select to attempt a personal best time. Perhaps the best advice is to ensure a period of acclimatization prior to the race.

Acclimatization

Acclimatization involves repeated exposure to exercise in the heat, which can be carried out in a hot climate (ideally where the marathon is to take place) or in a laboratory acclimatization chamber (correctly known as acclimation). The end result is the same, regardless of the method, namely that the runner has an increased tolerance to exercise in the heat. This is achieved by the runner beginning to sweat sooner and at a lower core temperature, in a greater volume and over a greater surface area. The sweat also has a lower salt content. As less sodium is lost, there is more in the body to help hold on to fluid that is ingested (*see* Chapter 3).

Runners may believe that fluid requirements will fall as they become acclimatized to the environmental conditions, but in fact the reverse is true. Heat acclimatization actually increases the requirement for fluid replacement because of the increased sweat losses.

Adaptation is normally complete after seven to fourteen consecutive days exercising in the heat, although it can take longer in some individuals. Low-volume training for sixty to ninety minutes is recommended for the first few days in the heat.

Exposure to Sun

Even a mild reddening of the skin can be uncomfortable and reduce acclimatization by damaging sweat glands. It may impair temperature regulation for up to ten days. A high factor, non-oily sunscreen should therefore be used before any exposure to sunlight. It should be applied thirty minutes before going out in the sun, to allow the skin to absorb some of it, and it should be reapplied regularly. Eyes should also be protected by wearing eye protection with a UV filter. Runners should also consider wearing a cap or hat as this will help to limit the heat load to the head. Any sunbathing should be delayed until after the marathon.

It may be an appealing idea to run a 'hot-weather' marathon, but non-elite runners should consider carefully whether they are making a wise choice. If they do decide to run they must allow themselves enough time to do all the things needed to minimize the risks of heat illness during the race, including the days needed to acclimatize completely before the marathon. Marathons run in these conditions can also be potentially dangerous, but it is now generally acknowledged that fun runs and shorter distances in the same conditions have an even greater potential to cause serious health problems. This is because the major factors causing heat stroke are the weather, running speed and individual susceptibility.

KEEPING UP YOUR FLUIDS

Runners will have to work at their fluid intake – nobody automatically drinks enough to prevent dehydration.

Ideally, runners should have a drinks bottle with them all the time (with something in it!), taking regular gulps.

Water or other suitable drinks should be drunk with all meals and if possible at the end of the meal as well. Extra salting at meals may be needed in the first days of acclimatization, particularly if sweat losses are high.

A variety of drinks – water, sports drinks, soft drinks, juices, and tea and coffee – can be drunk. Tea and coffee should not be drunk in greater amounts than usual.

Keeping a water bottle by the bed makes drinking in wakeful moments easier.

Sports drinks are ideal for use immediately before, during and after running. However, these drinks do have an energy value and if drunk all the time could cause unwanted weight gain.

CHAPTER 7
Running into Problems

The last thing a runner needs in their preparation for a marathon is a disruption to their training schedule through illness or injury. Sometimes this is unavoidable – such as an infectious disease picked up from a child or an accident at home or work – but in many cases enforced breaks in training through illness or injury can be avoided with a little more attention to diet, among other precautions. Problems that are often considered to be occupational hazards of running – muscle cramps, runner's trots and stitches – can often be prevented or at least minimized by making changes to the diet or eating patterns.

GASTROINTESTINAL SYMPTOMS

Gastrointestinal symptoms occur frequently in marathon runners, the commonest being nausea, vomiting, intestinal cramps and diarrhoea, as well as less severe complaints such as abdominal bloating, burping and flatulence.

Nausea and Vomiting

Pushing the body to the limits often results in nausea, vomiting and a decreased appetite during and for some time after exercise. There are several theories why this happens. One is that an abnormality develops in the way the nerves supply certain blood vessels in the brain and stomach, and this causes nausea and vomiting. In this case, reducing the level of exertion or effort

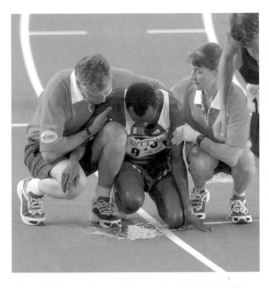

Ahmed Adam Saleh suffers at the IAAF World Championship Marathon in Edmonton. (EMPICS)

should get rid of these symptoms. However, problems may be due to mechanical effects as pressure builds up in the abdomen, which in turn causes a gastro-oesophageal reflux of the stomach contents. In other words, the stomach contents are forced back up the oesophagus into the mouth and removed from the body in a fairly undignified manner. Allowing a longer period of time between eating and running may provide the solution.

Gastric retention (stomach contents tending to hang around too long before they are released into the small intestine) has also been

126

suggested as a cause of this problem. However, it could simply reflect a tendency to motion sickness, in which case suitable medication from the doctor should remedy it. Finally, recent research now suggests that dehydration or high intakes of fat and protein may be common causes of exercise-induced nausea.

Runner's Trots

Many runners experience abdominal cramps, diarrhoea and the 'urge to go' during or immediately after running. Several causes for this inconvenient and often embarrassing side-effect of running have been suggested, including the bouncing action of running, a rise in certain hormones that increase bowel movements, a fall in blood flow to the intestines, particularly during more exacting runs, dietary reasons and, of course, race-day nerves. If the bowel is heavy with waste products, the running action may press the contents against the gut wall, causing fluid to be released into the gut. This can dilute the gut contents, make them more liquid, and so provoke a bout of diarrhoea.

The trots tend to occur in the later stages of long training runs or the marathon itself, often around the 20-mile mark (when less experienced runners may also be hitting the wall, as their carbohydrate stores become seriously depleted). Levels of the stress hormone cortisol rise at this time and as a result a runner may experience an overwhelming desire to stop running and rest. At the same time, parasympathetic nerves are stimulated by the release of cortisol, which leads to stimulation of the bowel. These effects alone surely provide a potent reason for a gradual increase in mileage, as well as the need for several good long runs under the belt before a complete marathon race is tackled.

Frequent digestive problems during or after running may be alleviated by switching training runs, when practical, from morning to evening, or vice versa. Runners who are troubled with the trots should try reducing their daily intake of high-fibre foods, for example, switching from wholemeal to white or brown bread, choosing a lower-fibre breakfast cereal (by comparing the nutritional information on the boxes), and certainly avoiding any foods with 'added fibre'. Particular care must be taken to have a low fibre intake the day before a race. It is sometimes possible to train an overactive gut to perform before rather than during a run. For instance, a possible routine before an early-morning run might be to get up and immediately make and drink a hot drink, then do all the necessary preparations, including warming up, before making a trip to the lavatory the very last thing before starting to run. Although the runner may be anxious to get out running, it is important to allow sufficient time to make the visit to the lavatory totally successful. With time, this can eventually become a regular pre-exercise habit, which will certainly be an advantage on the day of the marathon.

One other cause of this problem may be a mild food intolerance intensified by running. Experimenting by withdrawing a single food item for twenty-four hours or more will prove if this is the case. Milk is often cited as a cause of food intolerance but as this is such an important source of essential nutrients it is important to prove it is the culprit before excluding it long-term from the daily diet. If simple changes to the diet and dietary habits do not help, advice should be sought from a doctor.

If the trots are only an occasional problem, particularly associated with race days, taking a dose of Imodium (Ioperimide) the day before should help to control things, although it will not cure the problem. If symptoms get worse or occur more frequently, a visit to the GP should be made to clear up the problem once and for all.

Gassy Problems

The likely cause of excessive amounts of gas is the diet. Once food is digested and absorbed, colonies of bacteria in the large intestine or colon use the residue for a source of nutrients and produce gas or 'wind' as a by-product. Certain foods are more gas-producing than others and runners with this problem should avoid beans (including baked beans), cabbage, broccoli and Brussels sprouts, or indeed any other foods known to exacerbate it, particularly before a race.

General Dietary Advice

Increased amounts of protein, fat, fibre and hypertonic fluids are all factors that decrease stomach emptying, which, in turn, appears to be correlated with an increased prevalence of gastrointestinal problems. Dehydration and thermal stress also seem to have a negative effect on gastrointestinal functioning. Recommendations, particularly on race day, are therefore to drink sufficient non-hypertonic drinks to prevent dehydration and to have a carbohydrate-rich diet that is low in fibre, fat and protein. This will ensure that carbohydrate stores are topped up and hydration maintained, while at the same time minimizing the risk of gastrointestinal problems spoiling the race. Finally, simply changing eating habits may help some runners. For instance, eating more slowly and seated at a table (never standing up or slumped in a chair in front of the television) may be all that is needed to resolve a gut problem.

HAEMATURIA (BLOOD IN THE URINE)

Although it is a frightening symptom, in most cases haematuria is a harmless condition (also called foot strike haemolysis) caused by the constant pounding of feet on hard surfaces such as pavements. The red blood cells get broken up as the feet hit the ground and, if not filtered efficiently by the kidneys, end up being excreted in the urine. Wearing well-cushioned running shoes, minimizing running on hard roads and keeping well hydrated will help to cure and prevent the condition.

Blood in the urine that is accompanied by other symptoms, such as painful, frequent urination, an urgent need to urinate or difficulty in starting to urinate, could be due to an infection or other cause. Runners who pass blood in the urine should always be checked out by their doctor and never try to self-diagnose. A doctor can establish the cause and prescribe any necessary treatment. Runners who have experienced blood loss in this way should ensure that their diet contains plenty of well-absorbed iron to top up losses that will have occurred due to the haematuria. What might look like blood in the urine may be something as innocuous as the result of eating beetroot.

THE STITCH

The stitch (exercise-related transient abdominal pain, or ETAP) is a localized pain in the abdomen, particularly at the side. It is experienced at some time or another by an estimated 60 per cent of runners per year. It does not seem to discriminate between the sexes but it does seem to affect younger rather than older runners and appears to be more common when runners are going downhill. Sometimes, runners are able to carry on through a stitch but often it is necessary to slow down or even stop running completely. Although the pain usually stops quite quickly, a severe stitch can leave a runner with soreness for a day or two. A severe stitch produces a sharp or stabbing pain, whereas a less intense pain has a more cramping, aching or pulling feeling.

There are many theories about the reasons why it occurs, and it is quite possible that there is more than one cause. Many scientists used to believe that the cause was a lack of oxygen resulting from blood shunting away from the rib-cage area, and/or diminished blood flow due to excessive muscle contractions. Others believed it was the effect of food and fluid in the small intestine pulling on the ligaments attached to the diaphragm. More recent and plausible research suggests it is the parietal peritoneum, or lining of the whole abdominal wall, that causes the problem. This lining is very sensitive to movement when irritated, which is why stitch pain tends to go away quickly once running stops. Indeed, any pain arising from the parietal peritoneum is sharp and stabbing and the site is easily located. The stitch would appear to be no exception to this. When the irritation of the parietal peritoneum is under the diaphragm, it causes what is called 'shoulder-tip pain' – an aching or sharp pain, which, again, is often experienced by runners.

Runners who do get a stitch may find that just reducing their pace is sufficient to alleviate the problem. Others will have to stop running. Bending forward and breathing deeply while pressing the painful area quite hard usually helps to get rid of the stitch.

Irritation of the parietal peritoneum may be caused by friction on the membrane. Stomach bloating after eating or drinking, or distension of the large bowel may place more pressure on the parietal peritoneum, which sets up the friction-type response. Hypertonic drinks have been suggested as a specific cause, as they move more slowly through the stomach, resulting in a greater mass of fluid in the gut.

PRACTICAL WAYS TO AVOID THE STITCH

Wait two to four hours after a meal before running and particularly avoid running after a heavy meal to allow time for stomach contents to empty into the small intestine.

High-fat foods and very high-sugar foods and drinks should be avoided as they take longer to digest.

Be well hydrated before and during running to maintain hydration status. Drink little and often to prevent overstretching the stomach walls.

Avoid hypertonic drinks (fruit juices, soft drinks and hypertonic energy drinks) before and during exercise, as these empty slowly from the stomach, and a full stomach may contribute to the development of a stitch.

Drink small, regular volumes of isotonic or hypotonic sports drinks or water, whichever is most appropriate for a particular run.

Increase training load gradually, in terms of both duration and intensity.

MUSCLE CRAMPS

Cramps are painful but temporary involuntary muscular contractions or spasms, usually affecting the gastrocnemius (calf muscle), hamstrings (back of the thigh) or quadriceps (front of the thigh). Cramps often occur in runners who suddenly increase their speed, run a lot further than usual, or run on unfamiliar terrain. Working the muscles harder than usual or using different, weaker sets of muscles can cause an overload, early muscle fatigue and a possible build-up of lactic acid. For example, runners who have never run more than 18 miles before their first marathon may experience muscle cramps in the last few miles.

General advice for the susceptible runner is to allow plenty of rest and recovery time, particularly after hard sessions, do an adequate pre-race stretch concentrating on the vulnerable muscles, take on board adequate and appropriate fluids and carbohydrate before and during running, and not run too fast too soon.

Some runners also experience cramping in the arms, chest, shoulders and neck, particularly in the later stages of a marathon. This may be caused by poor posture as the runner tires, but weak upper-body strength is a more likely cause. Including some upper-body strength and conditioning work in the training programme, stretching the chest muscles and arms as a regular part of the warm-up, and being conscious about posture while running should all help to avoid upper-body cramping. Finally, wearing comfortable clothing and running shoes – so that the body is not constricted in any way – may also help.

Several minerals, including magnesium, potassium and calcium, have been implicated in causing muscle cramps. Gaining more credibility by the day, however, is the view that cramps, particularly those often referred to as heat cramps, can be related to muscle fatigue and loss of large amounts of both fluid and sodium all acting together. Sodium is an important mineral for correct functioning of nerves and muscles, and a shortage of sodium as well as fluid can make muscles more irritable and twitchy. Following healthy eating advice to cut back on salt intake, drinking water rather than a sports drink, and drinking in insufficient amounts may be some of the reasons why so many runners experience muscle cramps. Poor refuelling of muscle glycogen stores will also compound the problem. Runners susceptible to cramping, who are probably also those who start sweating early, those who sweat a lot and those whose sweat is particularly salty, may be able to cure the problem by using a sports drink rather than water and adding salt to their diet. However, the use of salt tablets is not usually recommended or necessary in marathons.

Muscle cramps should be treated by allowing the muscle to relax through stretching and massage, and the application of ice if the cramp is severe. Rest and fluid replacement are also key factors in recovery. Persistent, severe or regular cramping that is not helped by these treatments, or cramps that are not related to running should be checked out by a doctor.

PRACTICAL WAYS TO AVOID CRAMPS

Get fit, as cramps are less common in well-trained athletes.

Drink plenty of fluids to stay hydrated during training, particularly sports drinks that have adequate sodium contents.

Carry out the 'sweat test' regularly (in different weather conditions and training sessions) to ensure sufficient fluids are always being consumed (*see* Chapter 3).

Add salt to meals, particularly during hot weather when sweat losses are higher. Craving salty food should be taken as an indication that this is what the body needs. Healthy eating advice aimed at the unfit general public is not necessarily always appropriate for fit, active people training to run a marathon.

Ensure the diet contains plenty of fruit and vegetables.

Include carbohydrates at all meals and ensure adequate refuelling takes place after all training sessions.

Warm up and stretch before running and stretch again afterwards. Stretch before bed if night cramps are a problem.

Allow adequate recovery and rest after hard training sessions.

MUSCLE SORENESS

Muscle aches and pain are synonymous with marathon training. Like any exercise, running causes tiny little tears in muscles, which can lead to inflammation, tightness and stiffness. Runners suffer most when they are just starting a training programme or when they start to increase the weekly mileage. A good warm-up before running can boost the circulation and make the muscle work more efficiently. Studies have shown that a massage by a trained professional physiotherapist or masseur can reduce muscle soreness twenty-four to forty-eight hours after a long run. The massage helps to get rid of waste products that have accumulated in the muscles and also helps to identify and repair tiny muscle tears and adhesions.

Including plenty of foods rich in antioxidants may also help to reduce muscle damage and prevent inflammation. Fruits and vegetables not only contain the ACE or antioxidant vitamins, and some minerals that have antioxidant properties, but also an enormous range of protective phytochemicals (not found in vitamin and mineral supplements). The more colourful the choice of fruits and vegetables, the greater the range of antioxidants that will be achieved. Kiwis, apples, oranges, papayas, peppers, tomatoes and dark green vegetables such as broccoli and cabbage should be regulars on the shopping list – enough to provide between five and nine portions of fruit and vegetables a day. Particularly good sources of vitamin E are seeds, nuts, wheatgerm, wholemeal bread and cereals, green plants, milk and milk products, and egg yolks.

JOINT CARE

Running can put a burden on joints and neglecting joint care can lay the foundations for problems in years to come. Surveys of ex-elite sportsmen and women have confirmed an increased incidence of osteoarthritis (OA). OA is a degeneration of the joints in the body, often referred to as the 'wear and tear' arthritis, which commonly affects the hip and knee joints. It is particularly prevalent in practitioners of high-impact sports such as football, rugby, racket sports and running. However, research has shown that there is no difference between the joints and bones of recreational

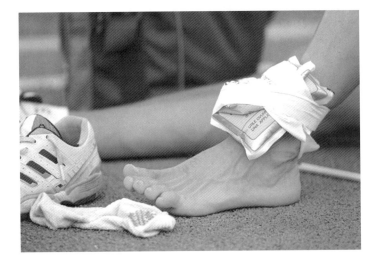

Treatment for a runner's injured ankle. (EMPICS)

runners and non-runners in later life. In fact, those who run an average three hours a week tend to have stronger bones and joints and a lower incidence of OA. Elite runners who have maintained a regular high mileage throughout their running career, and those who sustained a previous joint injury, however, have an increased risk of OA in later life compared with non-runners. Poor biomechanics is also believed to lead to premature OA in runners.

It is important not to see the possible negative effects of running in isolation but to take into account all the positives for both elite and non-elite runners: improved life expectancy, lower risk of heart disease and diabetes, and reduced incidence of obesity. The best advice should surely be to carry on running, but to take all available measures to protect the joints.

Injuries usually occur as a result of specific trauma to the muscle, bone or ligament, or repetitive micro-trauma or overuse of these structures, such as tendonitis. Injuries that occur directly to a joint or result in abnormal joint alignment and/or instability may lead to earlier degeneration of that joint. Often the cartilage (the shock absorber in joints) at the end of the bones is damaged and becomes irregular and thinner. This causes more stress to be put on the underlying bone, which in turn becomes thicker in response to increased compressive forces. The entire process of cartilage degeneration and subsequent bony changes is referred to as osteo- or degenerative arthritis.

The long-chain marine sources of omega-3 fatty acids can help care for joints and keep them supple and flexible. New research at the University of Cardiff in Wales suggests that they may also have a role in maintaining cartilage health, by halting or even reversing cartilage degeneration. Their anti-inflammatory properties can also help to relieve pain and stiffness. In theory, omega-3 fatty acids should be widely available from the diet but, despite all the encouragement to eat more oily fish, this

advice is not being heeded. Other sources of omega-3 fatty acids include walnuts, pumpkin seeds and linseed or flax oil, food items that may not be included in the diet on a regular basis. Taking a cod liver oil supplement containing these essential fatty acids is for many the preferred option, guaranteeing a regular daily intake in a controlled amount. For runners with memories of the nasty-tasting cod liver oil of the past, the good news is that modern cod liver oil supplements have no taste or smell, and do not repeat after being swallowed!

Glucosamine is a natural substance found in the body and made by the combination of glucose and the amino acid glutamine. It is found mainly in the cartilage, where it has an important role in keeping the cartilage healthy and resilient. Many researchers believe that joint cartilage is constantly rebuilding itself so that worn-out and damaged cartilage is always being replaced. Glucosamine has been shown to regenerate cartilage, plus it also appears to have anti-inflammatory effects. Findings from the majority of studies show that glucosamine supplementation provides some pain relief and improved function in people with regular knee pain. However, the benefits do not normally become apparent until regular supplementation has continued for at least six weeks. Available evidence suggests that a dose of 1,500mg a day of glucosamine sulphate is as good as non-steroidal anti-inflammatory drugs (such as Ibuprofen) in helping to relieve the symptoms of OA in the knee. When buying a glucosamine supplement it is important to check the label to make sure the product contains enough of the active ingredient (glucosamine sulphate) in the manufacturer's recommended daily dosage.

Vitamin C has many important functions in the body, one of which is in collagen formation. Collagen is a structural fibrous protein found in all connective tissues such as bones, cartilage, ligaments, tendons and skin. It is the most abundant protein in the body. One of the easiest ways of maintaining a good regular intake of vitamin C is to ensure that plenty of fresh fruit and vegetables are included in the daily diet. This will also help to supply other nutrients and biologically active substances such as flavonoids, which have not only antioxidant properties but also anti-inflammatory properties.

Chondroitin is another component of cartilage. It helps to attract fluid and nutrients into the cartilage, where the fluid acts like a spongy shock absorber, protecting existing cartilage from premature breakdown. Glucosamine and chondroitin work together to reduce the progression of OA after joint injury, prevent cartilage thinning due to OA, and improve pain and function in mild to moderate OA. Supplements containing cod liver oil, glucosamine and chondroitin are becoming more and more popular with athletes across many sports including running. They represent a simple and effective way of helping to preserve joints and keep them functioning properly and painlessly.

STRESS FRACTURES

Stress fractures occur in runners whose bones are too weak to cope with the load that running imposes on them. Females seem to be more prone to stress fractures than men and those with menstrual abnormalities are especially at risk. Most stress fractures occur in beginners (about eight to twelve weeks into their programme), or runners who suddenly increase their training load. There is evidence to indicate that those females with menstrual abnormalities have weaker bones, possibly because their intake of dietary calcium is too low to maintain normal bone mineral content. In this case, calcium intakes should be increased, although there is as yet no firm evidence that

this will reduce the risk of a recurrent injury. Major sources of calcium are milk, cheese, yoghurt, canned sardines and pilchards (as long as the bones, softened by the canning process, are eaten), dark green leafy vegetables, pulses, white flour and bread, and hard water.

THE COMMON COLD AND OTHER INFECTIONS

Who Is at Risk?

The common cold is a viral infection, caused by over 200 viruses, resulting in inflammation of the mucous membranes lining the nose and throat. Colds tend to occur in cold weather, as viruses thrive in these conditions. Cold viruses are carried through the air in droplets, making stuffy offices, trains and buses with closed windows and poorly ventilated areas notorious breeding grounds. The well-known symptoms include head and nasal congestion, sore throat, coughing, headache, sneezing and watery eyes. It is estimated that adults catch between two and five colds a year. Children generally get more because their immune systems have not yet developed and matured.

Research shows that runners are at greater risk of catching colds and other viruses in the first three hours after finishing a marathon, because their immune system has become suppressed. A recent study undertaken at the Los Angeles Marathon showed that one in seven runners was ill after the marathon and that those runners covering more than 95km (60 miles) a week in the two months before the race were twice as likely to be ill compared with those running fewer than 30km (20 miles) a week. However, another study has shown that regular moderate weekly mileage appears to have a protective influence, with runners having fewer colds than their sedentary peers. Upper respiratory tract infections (URTI) are also common during periods of hard training, although during less-intensive training periods runners have the same risk of picking up an infection as a less active person. Running to near exhaustion reduces the antibodies that help fight bacteria and viruses and this immune suppression can last for anything from three to seventy-two hours.

Cold Cures

The general advice is to keep up fluids, eat plenty of fruit (and, indeed, any foods that seem particularly appetizing), generally take things easy and dose with paracetamol or aspirin to lessen the symptoms. What else can a runner do to minimize the number of training days lost? It has been found that taking 500–1,000mg of vitamin C a day, from the time when cold symptoms first appear until they have gone, lessens the severity and possibly the duration of a cold. The benefits of taking such doses as a prophylactic have not been proven and there is no justification for taking such large doses of vitamin C on a regular basis.

In a study published in 2002, forty-eight patients recruited within twenty-four hours of developing cold symptoms were given a lozenge containing 12.8mg of zinc acetate or a placebo, every two to three hours while awake (about 80mg zinc, or nearly five times the RNI a day), for as long as they had cold symptoms. Overall, the average duration of cold symptoms was 4.5 days in those taking zinc, compared with 8.1 days in those on the placebo. The most significant reduction of a specific symptom was for coughing. Compared with the placebo, those taking zinc supplements suffered more from dry mouth and constipation but incidence of bad taste and mouth irritation was similar to the placebo group. The researchers suggest that this supplement regimen should not cause any problems but they do recommend that if there is

no clear improvement within three days, supplementation should be discontinued.

The herbal remedy echinachea is widely used to treat the common cold but at the moment there seems no clear consensus about its effectiveness. Runners who opt to use it should ensure they use an effective preparation (not all preparations are), manufactured by a reputable supplier. Some runners find garlic and chillies helpful in minimizing the effects of a cold. Runners with severe nasal congestion can also try adding a few drops of eucalyptus oil to a bowl of steaming water, covering their head with a towel and inhaling the steam deeply.

For colds and URTI above the neck, light exercise will actually speed recovery, as long as the exercise is very low in intensity – walking, jogging or light cycling are all appropriate. It is important for runners to be aware of how they feel and to appreciate that this is not the time to push themselves.

Influenza or flu, a much more serious viral infection, targets the upper and lower respiratory passages. Symptoms include headache, fever, muscular pain and weakness, and possibly joint pain, sensitivity to light, nausea and vomiting. Training is out of the question, but runners who succumb to flu are unlikely to be able to get out of bed. Runners should never attempt to sweat out a fever as this can exacerbate the condition and make recovery take longer.

DIET AND IMMUNE FUNCTION

Hard training is associated with reduced immune function. This effect is even more evident if a runner is following a particularly heavy training schedule on a poor diet. Runners are much more susceptible to infections if their diet is lacking in energy (particularly carbohydrate), protein, iron, zinc and vitamins A, E, B_6 and B_{12}. To maintain immune function, a diet

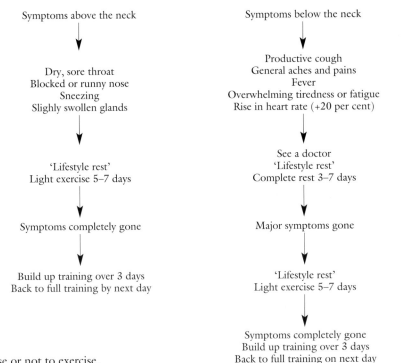

Symptoms above the neck

↓

Dry, sore throat
Blocked or runny nose
Sneezing
Slightly swollen glands

↓

'Lifestyle rest'
Light exercise 5–7 days

↓

Symptoms completely gone

↓

Build up training over 3 days
Back to full training by next day

Symptoms below the neck

↓

Productive cough
General aches and pains
Fever
Overwhelming tiredness or fatigue
Rise in heart rate (+20 per cent)

↓

See a doctor
'Lifestyle rest'
Complete rest 3–7 days

↓

Major symptoms gone

↓

'Lifestyle rest'
Light exercise 5–7 days

↓

Symptoms completely gone
Build up training over 3 days
Back to full training on next day

To exercise or not to exercise.

should be well balanced, meeting energy requirements and ensuring an adequate intake of carbohydrate, protein, vitamins and minerals. However, the use of megadosing with vitamins and minerals does not appear to be beneficial and, in fact, excess intakes can actually impair immune function. Adequate intakes of carbohydrate are essential, as poor intakes lead to depleted glycogen stores, increased levels of circulating stress hormones and a greater disturbance of several immune function indices. Consumption of 30–60g carbohydrate in drinks during prolonged exercise is recommended, as this does appear to help reduce some of the immunosuppressive effects of prolonged exercise. By keeping blood-glucose levels up, stress hormones are reduced and immune function is better maintained than when only water is drunk.

GLUTAMINE

Glutamine is an extremely abundant non-essential amino acid found particularly in skeletal muscle and plasma. It accounts for more than 60 per cent of the total intramuscular free amino acid pool. Glutamine is used primarily as a source of fuel by the gastrointestinal tract and the immune system. However, it is sometimes referred to as a conditional essential amino acid, because when the body is under stress (for example, following trauma or burns), the requirement for glutamine may not be met by body synthesis alone.

Although modest exercise stimulates immune function and protects against minor infections, hard or prolonged exercise can depress the immune system and increase the risk of illness. Some immune cells have been shown to use glutamine at a very high rate at this time, drawing on the supplies of glutamine in the plasma and consequently depleting them. This has led to the suggestion that oral supplementation with glutamine might help in maintaining plasma concentrations and that this, in turn, could possibly prevent the impaired immune function that follows prolonged exercise. Research to date does not appear to support this theory. The current view is that, although there is a fall in plasma glutamine level, it is not great, certainly compared with the fall that is observed in trauma and burns patients. The amount of glutamine present even after prolonged exercise is still believed to be sufficient for normal functioning of the immune cells. In other words, glutamine supplements are beneficial in the clinical setting but as yet have not been proven to be effective in getting rid of the post-exercise impairment of immune cell function. Nevertheless, glutamine is safe and has no apparent side-effects or health risks.

HOW TO AVOID ILLNESS

Ensure the diet contains plenty of fresh fruit and vegetables.

Include plenty of iron- and zinc-rich foods in the diet (*see* Chapter 1).

Maintain a high intake of carbohydrate-rich foods.

Avoid rapid weight loss – the diet is bound to be inadequate to support training.

Drink plenty of fluids that contain carbohydrate, before, during and after prolonged and intensive sessions. Not only do they maintain proper hydration, they can help lessen the stress on the immune system by blunting cortisol release (an immunosuppressive hormone) and reducing the post-exercise decrease in white blood cell function.

Allow plenty of rest and recovery time after training. Training is the stimulus to which the body adapts but adequate rest is required to allow time for the adaptations to take place. Include one or two rest days per week.

Keep a 'feelings' log on performance, mood, fatigue, muscle soreness and perception of effort. Reduce training load if normal training sessions appear harder than usual.

Aim for eight hours (but with a minimum of six hours) of quality sleep a night, with daytime naps if necessary.

Keep hands away from eyes and mouth.

Wash hands regularly, especially after touching anything previously touched by someone with a cold.

Avoid getting a dry mouth. Saliva has an anti-bacterial action so it is important to drink at regular intervals during the day. Maintain good oral hygiene.

Just before and immediately after running a race keep away from people who are poorly, young children and large crowds.

Avoid sharing food, cutlery and other utensils, particularly drinks bottles, with other people, especially other runners.

Use single-use wipes such as kitchen towels or disposable cloths in the kitchen. A recent study showed that after only one day's use in a domestic kitchen, the average reusable cloth contains over one billion germs.

Throw away food that is past its use-by-date, even if it looks and smells fine (*see* Chapter 2).

Have a vaccination against influenza.

UNEXPLAINED UNDERPERFORMANCE SYNDROME

Most runners will experience underperformance at some stage during training for a marathon but they will usually recover their form following a one- to two-week taper in training. Sometimes, this underperformance, usually accompanied by fatigue, continues for longer, despite resting for two weeks. This condition is believed to affect between 2 and 10 per cent of elite endurance athletes each year. No medical cause for the condition is found and it is now called 'unexplained underperformance syndrome' or UUPS; it was previously referred to variously as overtraining syndrome, burn-out and staleness. Runners may feel tired much of the time and complain about fatigue and heavy legs, but this is not seen as a problem, as such feelings are considered normal by those in hard training. On further questioning, however, runners may admit to other symptoms, including sleep disturbance, difficulty getting to sleep, nightmares, waking in the night, or alternatively 'enjoying' prolonged, uninterrupted sleep, but still not waking refreshed. They may complain of mood disturbances (with increased anxiety and irritability), loss of competitive drive, motivation, energy and libido. There may be loss of appetite and weight loss, lightheadedness and an increase in resting pulse rate. Runners may go down with minor infections, often getting a cold every three or four weeks.

There does not appear to be any medical cause for UUPS. Physiological, psychological, environmental and dietary stresses may all be partly to blame. Precipitating factors appear to be a sudden increase in training, stress of competition, and other 'outside' stresses, such as illness or injury, exams, moving house or relationship problems. Dietary stresses may be related to a negative energy balance, reduced carbohydrate intake, dehydration, micronutrient deficiencies (in vitamins, minerals and so on) and an amino acid imbalance. Whatever the cause, the end result is a reduction in immune function and an increased incidence of infections.

Regeneration strategies include relaxation, diet, fluids, reduction in stresses, regular sleep cycle and time for recovery. Many runners recover after six to twelve weeks, although it can take much longer. After a period of complete rest, light exercise is resumed using different regimes from normal training (in other words, not running), gradually building up

---

DIETARY MEASURES TO HELP PREVENT UUPS

Maintain an adequate energy intake to meet demands.

Make carbohydrate the major energy source.

Refuel adequately immediately after every training session.

Use a sports drink containing carbohydrate before, during and after all long training sessions. Apart from the direct effect that carbohydrate has in maintaining immune function, such drinks will maintain saliva flow rate. Saliva acts as a mechanical barrier against pathogens.

Keep up a good iron intake (non-red-meat eaters and vegetarians need to take particular care).

Ensure at least five portions of fruit and vegetables are eaten every day.

Eat and enjoy a wide variety of foods.

Try a warm drink of camomile tea before bed as this can help ensure good-quality sleep at night and may help to establish a more regular sleep pattern.

the duration and then the intensity. Recovery is monitored to prevent any recurrence of the condition.

FIT TO COMPETE

The 2002 publication *Road Races: Medical Aspects of Road Race Organization and Provision* (National Sports Medicine Institute of the United Kingdom and UK Athletics; ISBN: 0-9526657-2-7) provides advice about the safety and medical provision at road-race events. Although aimed primarily at the sport's governing body, event organizers and medical and paramedical personnel, it also gives recommendations for runners themselves. The following extract is reproduced with kind permission of the NSMI.

Considering your race entry
What factors should you consider before entering an event? Those who take part in regular physical activity or training will be less likely to have any cardiac or injury problems than those who do not. Have you trained or will you be able to train sufficiently for the event you are entering? Experience shows that some runners who had fatal cardiac problems during or soon after exercise have had symptoms in the preceding weeks or months but failed to seek medical advice. Have you had any symptoms of chest pain, rapid or irregular heartbeat, undue breathlessness? Have you ever passed out or fainted during exercise? Do you have any medical condition that might affect your ability to take part e.g. high blood pressure? Is there a strong family history of heart disease at an early age? If the answer to any of the above questions is 'yes', then you should consult your doctor for further advice or defer your entry.

The type of course and its hills and slopes will influence the effort you will require. A flat road race through familiar territory might be recommended for your first event. The time of year and likely weather conditions will also affect the stress on your body. Dehydration, cramps and collapse are more common during hot, humid conditions. A slow runner may struggle and become dangerously cold on a chilly damp day. Have you considered the course length, type and likely environmental conditions at the time of year?

Race day – still fit?
A lot can happen between placing your race entry and the event itself. Entrants who are fundraising for charities often feel under pressure to take part even if they are unwell or unfit because of the money they hope to raise. You should never run with a fever, as there is a risk of causing myocarditis (inflammation of the heart), which can be fatal or debilitating in the long term. Do not run if you feel unwell or have just been unwell. Most medical emergencies occur in people who have been unwell but do not wish to miss the race. If you feel feverish, have been vomiting, have had severe diarrhoea or any chest pains, or otherwise feel unwell, it is unfair to you, your family and the event support staff to risk becoming a medical emergency. You are unlikely to perform well and do yourself justice. There are many races but only one 'you'. If you are not fit then please withdraw from the event for your own safety.

Many entrants do have a past history of medical problems or will be taking medications or use inhalers. This information is invaluable to the medical support staff in the unlikely event that you collapse. For example, knowing that you are diabetic or asthmatic can speed the diagnosis and treatment of your problem. Please complete your medical details on the reverse of your race number. If you do not, it may prolong the time taken to give you the correct treatment.

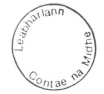

Dietitians in Sport and Exercise Nutrition (DISEN)

Dietitians in Sport and Exercise Nutrition (DISEN) is the name of the British Dietetic Association's Sports Nutrition Interest Group, which started in 1999. The British Dietetic Association (BDA) was formed in 1936 and incorporated in 1947. It is the professional association for qualified dietitians in the United Kingdom, and a condition of full membership is the holding of a recognized dietetic qualification

Members of DISEN are all professionally qualified dietitians who have undertaken further training in the specialist area of sports nutrition. Registered Dietitians work within the professional statement of conduct as laid down by The Health Professionals Council.

DISEN acts as a point of contact for information and support relating to sports nutrition for able-bodied and disabled athletes. A range of publications, including credit-card-sized laminated pee charts and A4 laminated pee chart posters and a Directory of Accredited Sports Dietitians are available. Publication and price lists or more information about the group can be obtained by writing to:

Dietitians in Sport and Exercise Nutrition
PO Box 22360
London
W13 9FL
www.disen.org

APPENDIX II
Useful Addresses and Websites

ADDRESSES

The British Dietetic Association
5th Floor, Charles House
148/9 Great Charles Street
Queensway
Birmingham
B3 3HT
www.bda.uk/com

British Nutrition Foundation
High Holborn House
52–54 High Holborn
London
WC1V 6RQ
www.nutrition.org.uk

British Olympic Association
1 Wandsworth Plain
London
SW18 1EH
www.boa.org.uk

British Paralympic Association
Norwich Union Building
9th Floor, 69 Park Lane
Croydon
Surrey
CR9 1BG
www.paralympics.org.uk

Dietitians in Sport and Exercise Nutrition
PO Box 22360
London
W13 9FL
www.disen.org

Eating Disorders Association
103 Prince of Wales Road
Norwich
NR1 1DW
www.edauk.com

Food Standards Agency
UK Office
Aviation House
125 Kingsway
London
WC2B 6NH
www.food.gov.uk
www.eatwell.gov.uk

The Nutrition Society
10 Cambridge Court
210 Shepherds Bush Road
London
W6 7NJ
www.nutritionsociety.org

Sports Council for Northern Ireland
House of Sport
Upper Malone Road
Belfast
BT9 5LA
www.sportni.net

Sports Council for Wales
Sophia Gardens
Cardiff
CF11 9SW
www.sports-council-wales.co.uk

Sport England
3rd Floor, Victoria House
Bloomsbury Square
London
WC1B 4SE
www.sportengland.org

Sport Scotland
Caledonia House
South Gyle
Edinburgh
EH12 9DQ
www.sportscotland.org.uk

UK Athletics
Athletics House
Central Boulevard
Blythe Valley Park
Solihull
West Midlands
B9D 8AJ
www.ukathletics.net

UK Sport
40 Bernard Street
London
WC1N 1ST
www.uksport.gov.uk

The Vegan Society
Donald Watson House
7 Battle Road
St Leonards on Sea
East Sussex
TN37 7AA
www.vegansociety.com

Vegetarian Society of the United Kingdom
Parkdale
Dunham Road
Altrincham
Cheshire
WA14 4QG
www.vegsoc.org

USEFUL WEBSITES

Active Places: www.activeplaces.com
American College of Sports Medicine: www.acsm.org
Association of International Marathons and Road Races: www.aims-association.org
Australian Institute of Sport: www.ais.org.au
British Masters Athletic Federation: www.bvaf.org.uk
*Consumer Lab*s (publish updated information on the purity of commercial products): www.consumerlabs.com
Gatorade Sports Science Institute: www.gssiweb.com
International Association of Athletics Federation: www.iaaf.org

London Marathon: www.london-marathon.co.uk
Lucozade Sport Science Academy: www.thelssa.com
UK Athletics Club Website Directory: www.runtrackdir.com/ukclubs
US Food and Drug Administration: www.fda.gov
Women's Running Network: www.womensrunningnetwork.co.uk
World Anti-Doping Agency: www.wada-ama.org

Dietetic Organizations

American Dietetic Association: www.eatright.org
American Sports, Cardiovascular and Wellness Nutritionists Dietetic Practice Group: www.scandpg.org

Australian Dietetic Association: www.daa.asn.au
Sports Dietitians Australia: www.sportsdietitians.com
Canadian Dietetic Association: www.dietitians.ca
New Zealand Dietetic Association: www.dietitians.org.nz
South African Dietetic Association: www.dietetics.co.za

Athletics National Governing Bodies

America: www.usatf.org
Australia: www.athletics.org.au
Canada: www.athleticscanada.com
New Zealand: www.athletics.org.nz
South Africa: www.athletics.org.za
United Kingdom: ukathletics.net

UK MAGAZINES

Athletics Weekly: www.athletics-weekly.com
Runners World: www.runnersworld.com
Running Fitness: www.running-fitness.com
The Coach: www.thecoach-online.co.uk

Index